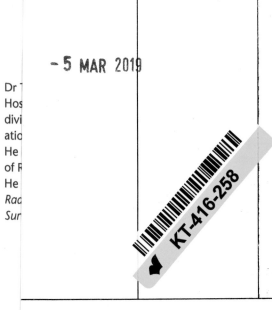 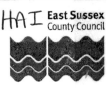

Overcoming Common Problems Series

Selected titles

A full list of titles is available from Sheldon Press,
36 Causton Street, London SW1P 4ST and on our website at
www.sheldonpress.co.uk

Overcoming Common Problems Series

Overcoming Common Problems Series

Overcoming Common Problems

Coping with Chemotherapy

Second edition

DR TERRY PRIESTMAN

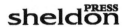

First published in Great Britain in 2005

Sheldon Press
36 Causton Street
London SW1P 4ST
www.sheldonpress.co.uk

Reprinted once
Second edition published 2009

The author and publisher have made every effort to ensure that the
external website and email addresses included in this book are correct and
up to date at the time of going to press. The author and publisher are not
responsible for the content, quality or continuing accessibility of the sites.

British Library Cataloguing-in-Publication Data
A catalogue record for this book is available from the British Library

ISBN 978-1-84709-080-5
eBook ISBN 978-1-84709-253-3

Typeset by Fakenham Prepress Solutions, Fakenham, Norfolk NR21 8NN
First printed in Great Britain by Ashford Colour Press
Subsequently digitally printed in Great Britain

Produced on paper from sustainable forests

Contents

Preface to the second edition

During the five years since the first edition of this book was published there have been a great many developments in the field of cancer chemotherapy. A key change has been the appearance of more new drugs that can specifically identify and attack cancer cells, causing relatively little damage to normal tissues. These are called targeted therapies and they generally have fewer and less severe side effects than the cytotoxic drugs (that interfere with cell division in both normal and cancer cells), which have formed the core of cancer chemotherapy for the past 60 years. In addition, results from recent clinical trials have confirmed the importance of a number of the newer hormonal drugs introduced for the treatment of breast cancer (which is now the commonest cancer in the UK) and prostate cancer (the commonest cancer in men). So an update of the text to reflect this progress was timely. Unfortunately, in the wider world beyond oncology, the worsening economic picture has focused attention on money matters, and so the section of the book dealing with the financial impact of cancer and chemotherapy has been expanded to give more advice on this subject.

Introduction

Every year in the UK nearly 200,000 people discover that they have cancer. Overall, about one in three of us can expect to develop cancer at some time during our lives. The good news to set against these depressing figures, though, is that over the past 30 years the outlook for people with most types of cancer has greatly improved. Complete cures are now possible for many cancers and, even when the condition is incurable, treatment can often offer many years of good-quality life before the illness reaches its terminal stage.

Chemotherapy plays a major role in cancer treatment and has transformed the outlook for many types of cancer over the past few decades. Very often, cures are now possible that could never have been imagined in the 1950s and 1960s. These days, at least half of all people who are diagnosed with cancer are likely to have some form of chemotherapy, at some time, during their illness.

Although chemotherapy has led to a large rise in the number of people being permanently cured, and considerable increases in life expectancy for many other people where cure was not possible, the word 'chemotherapy' still usually causes great anxiety and distress when it is first mentioned as being part of someone's treatment. To most people it means months of upsetting side effects, with a devastating impact on their day-to-day life. But although it can be very traumatic and disruptive, many people find that when they actually get started on treatment it is not nearly as bad as they had expected, and they are able to cope with it remarkably well. The reality of chemotherapy is often far less unpleasant than people imagine.

Much of the fear about chemotherapy comes from not really knowing what to expect, what will happen, or what to do when things do happen. These days, if you are going to have chemotherapy, then you are likely to be given lots of information about your treatment. But often this is passed on verbally by doctors or nurses in busy clinics, where it is difficult to take in, and it can also be hard to ask questions if there are things you don't understand. Even if you are given leaflets or booklets to back up what has been said at the hospital, these may only cover some aspects of your treatment or be written in a way that is difficult to understand – or you may feel that it just doesn't apply to you.

The aim of this book is to try to fill in the background about what chemotherapy is, what it does and how to carry on with life during and after your treatment. As the book is designed to cover the whole subject, only bits of it are likely to apply to your own situation, and so it is probably something that you will find more helpful to dip into and out of, rather than reading from cover to cover. It is not intended to replace information that you may be given at hospital, but to be used alongside it – perhaps to fill in some gaps, to give additional reassurance or to help you understand things by having them explained in a slightly different way.

Many people say that being aware of what is going on, understanding what to expect and knowing what to do when and if problems crop up makes coping with their treatment much easier. Being informed can greatly reduce the anxieties and uncertainties of chemotherapy, and can give you more control over what is happening to you.

1

What is chemotherapy?

The word 'chemotherapy' was first used by doctors to describe the use of drugs, like antibiotics, which were given to treat infections. When, about 60 years ago, the first drugs were discovered that could be given to treat cancer, the term was extended to include the use of these new compounds. In recent years people have become much more aware of drug treatment for cancer – partly because of its considerable success in increasing the number of cures, which means that more people than ever are having the treatment, and partly because of the sometimes distressing side effects that it can cause. With this growing public awareness the word 'chemotherapy' has increasingly come to be shorthand for 'cancer chemotherapy', and its original, broader meaning has largely been lost.

What is cancer?

Before going any further, it is important to be clear about what we mean by cancer.

We all begin our lives as a single cell fertilized in our mother's womb. That cell then divides to form two cells, those two cells divide to make four, and this process of cell division continues throughout pregnancy, and on through infancy, childhood and adolescence to produce the countless billions of cells that make up our adult selves.

Even in adulthood the process of cell growth continues, because cells are constantly wearing out and dying and need to be replaced. For example, the bone marrow, which produces the red cells, white cells and platelets that make up our blood, makes many millions of new cells every day to replace those that have worn out. Similarly, the cells that line parts of our digestive system are replaced every 24–48 hours.

Throughout our lives these processes of cell division and growth are very precisely controlled, so that we make exactly the number of new cells that our bodies need, no more and no less.

A cancer develops when the cells in a particular organ escape from these controls and begin to reproduce and grow in a haphazard way, producing more cells than they should. Over time these cells build up to form a tumour, or growth. If this is not treated, then the growth will begin to invade and destroy the tissue surrounding it. It may also send off seedlings – tiny clumps of cells – that spread to form secondary growths in other parts of the body. These seedlings may be carried either in the blood stream, or through the lymph vessels – the network of thread-like channels that drain fluid from the tissues into lymph glands (lymph nodes).

Tumours can be divided into two main types: benign and malignant. Benign tumours may grow to a large size but they do not actually invade and destroy the tissue surrounding them, and they do not spread to other parts of the body. Malignant tumours are able both to invade and destroy nearby tissue, and to form secondary growths. The word 'cancer' only applies to these growths; a benign tumour is not a cancer, but a malignant tumour is.

Most cancers start as a single growth in one part of the body; this is called the primary cancer. As it continues to grow, the primary cancer may, or may not, produce secondary cancers elsewhere. Another name for these secondary cancers is metastases. When a doctor or nurse talks about metastatic cancer, they mean a cancer that has already spread to other parts of the body.

Types of chemotherapy

There is an increasing number of different types of drug treatment that can be used to treat cancer.

The first of these to be developed is known as cytotoxic chemotherapy. Cytotoxic drugs are, as their name suggests, cell poisons. They work by damaging the cancer cell so that it is unable to divide and reproduce, and so it dies. Today there are more than a hundred different cytotoxic drugs that can be used in the treatment of cancer. Unfortunately, none of these drugs is able to tell the difference between cancer cells and normal cells. This means that when they are given they will cause some damage to normal cells as well as killing off the cancer cells, and this is why they can cause side effects.

The great majority of people prescribed drugs as part of their cancer treatment will be given cytotoxics. Because of this, when we talk about chemotherapy today, what we usually mean is cytotoxic chemotherapy.

Another type of drug treatment for cancer, developed at about the same time as cytotoxic drugs first appeared, is hormonal treatment. Hormonal therapy is only suitable for a very few types of cancer, but it does play an important role in the treatment of two very common conditions: breast cancer and prostate cancer. Hormonal drugs work very differently to cytotoxics and they generally cause fewer side effects.

More recently, other types of compounds have been discovered that can help in cancer treatment. Many of these are the so-called targeted drugs. These are compounds that attack specific abnormalities on cancer cells that are not present on normal cells. This means that – in contrast to the cytotoxic drugs – they only interfere with the growth of the cancerous cells, leaving normal cell growth virtually unaffected, so they are 'targeted' to the cancer. Not only are these newer drugs proving increasingly effective in cancer treatment but also they usually have less severe side effects than the more established cytotoxic drugs. The targeted therapies may be used on their own or given along with cytotoxic drugs or hormonal treatments.

Understandably, many people are often not sure exactly what type of chemotherapy they are having. Table 1 lists the drugs that are most often used in cancer chemotherapy and shows whether they are cytotoxic, hormonal or targeted treatments. More information about the different kinds of drugs is given in Chapter 3.

Table 1 Drugs commonly used in cancer chemotherapy

Class of drug	Drug name	Trade name(s) (where applicable)
Cytotoxic	bleomycin	
	busulfan	Myleran, Busilvex
	capecitabine	Xeloda
	carboplatin	Paraplatin
	carmustine, BCNU	BiCNU, Gliadel wafers
	chlorambucil	Leukeran
	cisplatin	
	cyclophosphamide	Endoxana
	cytarabine	
	dacarbazine, DTIC	
	dactinomycin, actinomycin D	Cosmegen Lyovac
	daunorubicin	
	docetaxel	Taxotere
	doxorubicin	Adriamycin
	epirubicin	Pharmorubicin
	etoposide	Etopophos, Vepesid
	fludarabine	Fludara
	fluorouracil	Efudix (topical)
	gemcitabine	Gemzar
	ifosfamide	Mitoxana
	irinotecan	Campto
	lomustine, CCNU	Lomustine
	melphalan	Alkeran
	mercaptopurine	Puri-Nethol
	methotrexate	
	mitomycin	
	mitoxantrone	
	oxaliplatin	Eloxatin
	paclitaxel	Paclitaxel, Taxol
	pemetrexed	Alimta
	procarbazine	
	raltitrexed	Tomudex
	temozolomide	Temodal
	thioguanine, tioguanine	Lanvis
	topotecan	Hycamtin
	vinblastine	Velbe
	vincristine	Oncovin
	vindesine	Eldisine
	vinorelbine	Navelbine

Class of drug	Drug name	Trade name(s) (where applicable)
Hormonal	anastrozole	Arimidex
	bicalutamide	Casodex
	buserelin	Suprefact
	cyproterone acetate	Cyprostat
	exemestane	Aromasin
	flutamide	Drogenil
	fulvestrant	Faslodex
	goserelin	Zoladex
	letrozole	Femara
	leuprorelin	Prostap
	medroxyprogesterone	Farlutal, Provera, Depo-Provera
	megestrol acetate	Megace
	norethisterone	
	stilboestrol	Diethylstilboestrol
	tamoxifen	Nolvadex-D
	triptorelin	Decapeptyl, Gonapeptyl
Targeted	alemtuzumab	MabCampath
	bevacizumab	Avastin
	bortezomib	Velcade
	cetuximab	Erbitux
	erlotinib	Tarceva
	gefitinib	Iressa
	imatinib	Glivec
	lapatinib	Tyverb
	nilotinib	Tasigna
	rituximab	MabThera
	sorafenib	Nexavar
	sunitinib	Sutent
	temsirolimus	Torisel
	trastuzumab	Herceptin

Chemotherapy and radiotherapy

Chemotherapy and radiotherapy are both important types of cancer treatment. People sometimes confuse them but they are very different. Chemotherapy relies on drugs, whereas radiotherapy uses high-energy, ionizing radiation to kill cancer cells.

Most radiotherapy treatments are given using machines called linear accelerators (or 'LinAcs' for short). The LinAc produces a beam of very high energy x-rays that can be focused on the part of the body where the cancer is. The patient lies on a couch by the machine for a few minutes for each treatment. The treatment itself is completely painless. Depending on the type of cancer, and the reason for the treatment, a course of radiotherapy can last anywhere from a single dose to 30–40 doses over six to eight weeks.

An important difference between radiotherapy and chemotherapy is that radiotherapy is a local treatment. It is only given to a particular part of the body where the cancer is – or might be – and so it only affects that area. With chemotherapy, the drugs that are used pass into the blood stream and will reach almost all parts of the body, and so it is a general, or – to use the medical word – a 'systemic' treatment. For more details, see *Coping with Radiotherapy* by Dr Terry Priestman (Sheldon Press, 2007).

A short history of cancer chemotherapy

Cytotoxic chemotherapy has its origins in the First World War, when mustine gas was used as a chemical weapon. One of the many toxic effects of the gas was to reduce dramatically the number of white blood cells in the body, leading to severe infections.

During the Second World War two American doctors, Louis Goodman and Alfred Gilman, working at Yale University realized that although the effect of mustine on the troops' white blood cells had been disastrous, there were illnesses in which such an effect might actually be beneficial. Leukaemias and lymphomas are types of cancer where the main problem is overproduction of white blood cells. They reasoned that if they could inject people who had leukaemia and lymphoma with small doses of mustine, then it might lower their numbers of white blood cells and help to control their illness. In 1942 they began some experiments on volunteers with these cancers, and discovered that, for a time at least, they could improve these patients' condition. So mustine was suddenly transformed from an agent of biological warfare to the first anti-cancer cytotoxic drug, and this ushered in the age of cancer chemotherapy.

The origins of hormonal therapy go back to the end of the

nineteenth century when, in 1896, a Glasgow surgeon called George Beatson published a report in the *Lancet* describing how he had treated a number of young women with advanced breast cancer by operating to remove their ovaries. He discovered that in some cases the cancers shrank quite remarkably for a period of time. In a parallel study the surgeon Charles Huggins, working in Chicago, reported in the 1940s that castration (surgically removing the testicles) of men with advanced prostate cancer often brought about an improvement in their condition. These observations were explained in the 1950s when a scientist called Elwood Jensen found that many breast and prostate cancer cells carried proteins called receptors that were stimulated by the female hormone oestrogen or the male hormone testosterone. As a result of these various studies, a number of drugs were developed that could interfere with the interaction between circulating sex hormones and the receptors on cancer cells, causing the cells to stop dividing and die off.

From the 1970s onward a number of other cellular systems have been discovered in which chemicals circulating in the blood, known as growth factors, stimulate receptors on cancer cells, causing them to grow and multiply. The identification of these processes has allowed scientists to develop drugs that can interfere with the receptors, making them inactive and so stopping cancer cell growth. In this situation the receptors are either only found on cancer cells or found in far greater quantities in the cancer cells than in normal cells (the technical term for this is 'over-expression' of the receptors). This means that the drugs only attack cancer cells, in contrast to the older cytotoxic drugs, which attack the process of cell division in both normal and cancer cells. This has led to these newer drugs being known as targeted therapies, because they are specifically aimed at cancer cells.

If we have so many drugs that attack cancer, why hasn't everyone been cured and why are we still looking for new drugs? The first thing to say is that for many types of cancer the outlook has been transformed by developments in chemotherapy over the past 50 years. Many conditions that in the 1950s and 1960s were almost always fatal can now almost always be cured. Unfortunately, however, this isn't universally true, and some cancers do remain a challenge. This is partly because different types of cancer respond differently to the drugs we have available – a treatment that works very well in one tumour type will often be completely ineffective in another. It is also the case that in some growths that appear to be sensitive to the treatment at first, resistant cancer cells will develop that are immune to the effects of drug treatment and will continue to grow and cause problems.

So we are still looking for the 'miracle cure', the 'wonder drug' or the 'magic bullet' that will provide the final answer for cancer treatment. The search goes on, and new drugs are being discovered all the time. But in parallel with this process of drug development, a better understanding of how to use the treatments we already have has also helped to improve results over the years.

How we use chemotherapy

When the first cytotoxic drugs appeared in the 1940s they were a completely novel form of treatment, and no one was sure how to use them.

At first doctors turned to the principles of antibiotic therapy, which had been established a few years before, as a guide. These suggested that just a single drug should be used, and it should be given sufficiently often to keep a fairly constant level of the drug in the blood at all times. With cytotoxics, the actual dose of the drug given was limited by its side effects and was adjusted to prevent these becoming too troublesome. This practice of giving one drug on a regular basis was called 'single agent continuous therapy'. Single agent continuous therapy did have some limited success in the 1950s, producing temporary improvements, but only temporary, in some advanced cancers, and actually leading to cures in two rare forms of cancer, namely Burkitt's lymphoma (an uncommon type of cancer of the lymph glands) and choriocarcinoma (a cancer affecting the womb, which occurs as a very rare complication of pregnancy). But in the common cancers this new drug treatment had very little impact.

By the 1960s, with more drugs available, doctors realized that different cytotoxics could affect the process of cell division in different ways. This led to the idea of giving two, or more, drugs at the same time, in the hope that by combining their different modes of action they would increase the number of cancer cells killed. This multiple drug continuous therapy was only briefly used because it was rapidly found that, although it did increase the damage to some cancers, it had a dramatic effect on the toxicity of treatment, causing very severe, sometimes lethal, side effects.

The breakthrough in overcoming this problem was the realization that normal cells were much better, and much quicker, at repairing the damage caused by chemotherapy drugs than cancer cells. This led to the suggestion, in the late 1960s, that it would be better to give the drugs as intermittent courses, or cycles, with a rest interval with no treatment in between, rather than giving them continuously. The idea underpinning this was that during the rest interval between courses the normal cells would be able to recover completely from any damage caused by the drugs, while the cancer cells would still not have made good the harmful effects of the previous course. The next course would then damage the cancer cells still further. In this way a number of courses could be given, with normal cells bouncing back between each cycle, while cancer cells were progressively killed off, until they had disappeared completely. This was called 'intermittent combination cytotoxic chemotherapy'.

Intermittent combination chemotherapy revolutionized cancer treatment and led to dramatic improvements in cure rates, or increased survival times, in many types of cancer during the 1970s and beyond. It is still the principle underpinning the use of cytotoxic chemotherapy today. By contrast, because they have little effect on the growth of normal cells, hormonal drugs and the newer targeted therapies do not usually have to be given intermittently, with periods for recovery, but are prescribed more like other drugs, being given on a daily, or sometimes weekly, basis.

Another major development that occurred during the 1970s and 1980s was the introduction of the use of drug treatment in early stages of the disease. Up until then chemotherapy had usually only been given to people with advanced cancer, which had spread widely throughout the body. Very occasionally, in a few types of cancer, this could bring about a cure, but usually all that happened was that the growth would shrink, or possibly even disappear, for a time, but then start growing again and still be ultimately incurable.

It was then suggested that in some types of cancer there might be a benefit in giving chemotherapy much earlier, immediately after initial surgical treatment to remove the primary tumour, with the hope being that this would prevent secondary cancers developing in the first place, rather than waiting for them to appear before starting the drug treatment. This idea of giving chemotherapy as an insurance policy to protect against the cancer coming back is called 'adjuvant chemotherapy'. The introduction of adjuvant chemotherapy has increased cure rates in a number of major cancers over the past 20 years, including breast cancer, lung cancer and bowel cancer.

2

Who needs chemotherapy?

Some basic facts about cancer

One in three to one in four of us will develop a cancer at some time during our lives. There are more than 200 different types of cancer that can affect our bodies. Some cancers are very common, whereas others are very uncommon. For example, each year in Britain about 40,000 people are diagnosed with lung cancer, but cancer of the heart is virtually unknown; similarly, although there are about 35,000 new cases of cancer of the large bowel (the colon and rectum) each year, only a handful of cancers of the small bowel are discovered. Some cancers grow very rapidly – certain forms of acute leukaemia and some types of lung cancer can be fatal within a few weeks if they are not treated. In contrast, others progress extremely slowly – some chronic leukaemias, and prostate cancer in older men, can often go for years without needing treatment or causing any problems. Some cancers, such as breast cancers and cancers of the kidney have a strong tendency to spread to other parts of the body, whereas others, such as rodent ulcers of the skin, hardly ever give rise to secondary cancers. Some cancers cause symptoms and are diagnosed at a very early stage in their development, for example cancers of the vocal cord, which cause hoarseness of the voice. Others often only cause problems when they have reached a more advanced stage, and so they are diagnosed much later in their development – this is often the case with cancers of the pancreas and the ovary.

About four out of every five cancers develop in cells that form the lining of the various organs of our bodies. These cells are called epithelial cells, and a cancer of the epithelial cells is called a carcinoma. So a carcinoma of the stomach is a cancer of the epithelial cells that form the inner lining of the stomach. Cancers of the supportive tissues of our bodies – the bones, muscles, fatty tissue and cartilage – are much less common, making up fewer than one in 20 cancers. These cancers of supportive tissue are called sarcomas. So a sarcoma of the stomach is a cancer of the muscular wall of that organ.

Both carcinomas and sarcomas typically begin as a single growth, the primary cancer, in a single organ, which may then spread to form secondary cancers in other parts of the body at a later time. By contrast, the other two major groups of cancers, the lymphomas and leukaemias, which make up about one in eight cancers, usually affect multiple sites throughout the body from their outset.

Lymphomas are cancers that arise in the lymph nodes or in patches of lymphatic tissue, which can be found in many of our body's organs. Leukaemias develop in the bone marrow and can also affect the lymph nodes and other organs.

Clearly then, cancers are a very diverse group of illnesses, and so very different approaches to treatment are needed for different types of cancer.

Cancer treatment

With such a spectrum of diseases, the treatment that is needed varies enormously depending on the particular type of cancer. In broad terms there are three main approaches to treatment: surgery, radiotherapy and drugs.

Surgery is still the cornerstone of treatment for most cancers, and it still accounts for the majority of cures. When dealing with carcinomas and sarcomas, provided that the primary growth has not become too large or spread to form metastases in other places, an operation to remove the growth has a good chance of curing the condition. Although surgery is very often curative, it may fail for one of two reasons: because microscopic traces of tumour, which would have been invisible to the surgeon, have been left behind; or because, again at a level too small to be detected, minute seedlings of the growth have already spread to form secondary cancers elsewhere.

Radiotherapy is often given after surgery to guard against the possibility of traces of cancer being left behind at the site of the operation. For example, in breast cancer, removing the primary tumour – either with a mastectomy, which takes the whole breast away, or a more conservative operation like a lumpectomy or wide local excision – apparently gets rid of the primary tumour. But if nothing more is done, then during the months or years after surgery microscopic remnants of the cancer that were missed will grow to form a local recurrence of the disease in about three out of ten people. Giving radiotherapy to the area after surgery is a way to reduce this risk, and it lowers the chances of local recurrence very dramatically. Radiotherapy is very often used in this way, as an adjunct to surgery, to reduce the risk of the tumour coming back. One advantage of radiotherapy is that it can safely cover a wider volume of tissue than can be removed at an operation, and so it can include the microscopic strands of cancer that may have spread into the normal tissue surrounding the primary growth, which would have been invisible at the time of the operation. In other situations radiotherapy may actually be used as an alternative to surgery as a curative treatment in its own right. It also has an important role to play in the more advanced stages of many cancers, when it can help in easing distressing symptoms such as pain, bleeding and breathlessness.

Although drug treatment has always been the mainstay of therapy for cancers such as lymphomas and leukaemias (and often results in a cure), for many years chemotherapy was only used in the treatment of the more advanced stages of carcinomas and sarcomas. Here it often was, and still is, successful in shrinking the disease, sometimes even making it disappear for a while, and increasing life expectancy, but almost inevitably the cancer would come back at some future time. In more recent years it has been used increasingly in the earlier stages of cancer, alongside surgery and/or radiotherapy, increasing the chances of a cure. This latter approach is known as adjuvant chemotherapy, and because many people find it rather difficult to understand it is worth a little more explanation.

Adjuvant chemotherapy

Adjuvant chemotherapy has been most widely used in breast cancer, and using this condition as an example is probably the easiest way to explain how it works.

Although surgery and radiotherapy will cure many women of their breast cancers, some women who appear to have been cured will return, months or years later, with the discovery of signs of spread of the disease to other parts of the body, such as the bones, liver, lungs or brain. These secondary cancers must have been present, as microscopic, undetectable seedlings of tumour, before the primary cancer was removed. The primary cancer could not have sent off metastases to other parts of the body after it had been taken away. The fact that these minute secondaries were missed when the original treatment was carried out was not a mistake by the doctors at the time – it was simply that whatever examinations, blood tests, x-rays or scans had been done, the tumours would have been too small to show up.

By the early 1970s the introduction of intermittent combination cytotoxic hemotherapy, giving three or more drugs together in cycles, or pulses, with rest periods in between for normal tissues to recover, had proved very effective in the more advanced stages of breast cancer, when the disease was extensive and incurable. The drugs would often reduce the size and number of the secondary cancers, relieve unpleasant symptoms and regularly extend survival, although they would not bring about a permanent cure. At the same time a new hormonal drug, tamoxifen, was discovered, which also helped to control advanced breast cancer.

As a result of these developments in treatment doctors began to wonder whether giving cytotoxic chemotherapy or tamoxifen, or both, to women who had apparently been cured by surgery and radiotherapy might completely kill off any microscopic seedlings of tumour that had spread elsewhere, and so increase their chance of a long-term cure.

In theory this was a good idea, but one problem was that not everyone who had surgery and radiotherapy for their early breast cancer would need the drugs; some women would have been truly cured by this treatment, whereas others would only appear to have been cured and would be at risk. But because the secondary cancers that posed that risk were too small to be detected, how could doctors know who did or did not need the drugs?

The answer was to find some feature of the cancer that suggested that a woman might be more at risk of harbouring those tiny seedlings of tumour spread. Doctors turned to statistics. These suggested that if the results of the initial surgery showed that the cancer had spread to one or more of the nearby lymph glands under the arm, on the same side as the affected breast, then – even if those nodes were removed completely – there was a greater likelihood that undetectable secondaries would be present in other sites than if the glands had all been completely free of tumour.

In the mid-1970s clinical trials began, in which women who had surgery to remove their breast cancer, but who were found to have one or more nearby lymph nodes involved with the cancer, were either given chemotherapy or tamoxifen, or both, or no further treatment. The results soon showed that the women who received the drug therapy had a much better chance of cure, and giving the additional treatment rapidly became standard practice.

Since then trials have continued, and are ongoing, to work out as precisely as possible who actually needs the treatment, and what is the best combination of drugs for each individual patient.

With time this principle of adjuvant, or precautionary, chemotherapy has also been extended to other types of cancer; it has proved valuable in bowel cancer, lung cancer, ovarian cancer and a number of other tumour types. Incidentally, although adjuvant chemotherapy is usually given after surgery, it is occasionally used before an operation is carried out and this is referred to as 'neo-adjuvant' therapy.

Although it can greatly improve someone's chance of a cure, with certain types of cancer there are at least two aspects of this adjuvant therapy that people often find hard to understand. The first is that, having had their initial surgery and/or radiotherapy, many people feel completely well. Therefore, because they have no apparent signs or symptoms of cancer, these patients find it difficult to accept that they may need extra treatment that can often go on for many months, and may cause troublesome side effects. Furthermore, even when all that treatment is complete, there is no way of telling whether it has been successful. Because there was no detectable or measurable cancer in the first place, there is no test that can be done at the end of the treatment to see whether those microscopic remnants of the disease, which may or may not have been present, were destroyed. Unfortunately, some people may need to wait some years to be sure that the cancer has been completely cleared from their bodies.

So who needs chemotherapy?

For many people with cancer, surgery, radiotherapy or a combination of the two will result in a cure, and they will not need any further treatment. But chemotherapy may be needed in the following situations.

- It may be the best first line of treatment to cure or control certain types of cancer. This is most likely to be the case in cancers such as lymphomas and leukaemias.
- It may be a wise precaution following surgery and/or radiotherapy in certain types of cancer to maximize the chance of cure and minimize the risk of the cancer coming back (adjuvant treatment).
- It may given in the more advanced stages of some cancers, occasionally in the hope of achieving a cure, but more often with the intention of controlling the disease, relieving symptoms and increasing life expectancy.
- It may be used to shrink the size of a cancer before surgery or radiotherapy is given (neo-adjuvant therapy).

3

Which drugs are used in chemotherapy?

There are more than 100 different drugs available for use in modern cancer treatment. The majority of these are cytotoxic agents, but hormonal therapies play a major role in the treatment of breast and prostate cancer, and the newer targeted therapies are becoming increasingly important in a wide range of cancer types. Some drugs are much more widely used than others, and this chapter mentions a few of the most important compounds.

Before going any further, a few words of explanation about drug names might be a good idea. Rather confusingly, most drugs in the UK have two names: a non-proprietary or proper name, and a proprietary or brand name. The non-proprietary name is the scientific name of the particular compound. The proprietary name is the trade name of the drug that has been patented by the company that makes it. Non-proprietary names are always written with the first letter in lower case; for proprietary names the first letter is always a capital. So, for example, Taxol is the trade name of the drug paclitaxel, and Campto is the trade name of the drug irinotecan. This means that during your treatment you might hear the same drug being talked about with two different names. With older drugs, for which the original manufacturer's patents have expired, often only the non-proprietary name is used. In this chapter if a drug has a commonly used brand name it is given in brackets after its non-proprietary name.

The cytotoxic drugs

The cytotoxic drugs have been grouped together in different families, based on their different ways of interfering with the process of cell division. Before describing these, a few words about the way in which cells divide might be helpful.

Cell division

Both normal cells and cancer cells are made up of a nucleus surrounded by a layer of cytoplasm. The nucleus contains the genetic material that determines how that cell will behave. This genetic information is carried in the genes. These genes are strung out along the chromosomes, a bit like pearls on a necklace. Each nucleus contains 23 pairs of these chromosomes.

The genes are made up of a protein called DNA. The DNA is made up of two strands of chemicals, twisted around one another in a spiral. When the cell is getting ready to reproduce and divide into two, it makes sufficient new DNA to form a complete new set of genes and chromosomes.

When this has been completed, the wall of the nucleus dissolves and the two sets of chromosomes separate to opposite sides of the cell, moving along a grid of fine tubes called the cell spindle. Once the separation of the two sets of chromosomes is complete the cytoplasm divides around them and the two new cells are created.

This process of cell division is called 'mitosis'.

The major families of cytotoxic drugs

Alkylating agents

The first cytotoxic to be discovered, mustine, was an alkylating agent. It is little used nowadays but a number of related compounds are still important. Two of these are cyclophosphamide, which is used to treat many different cancers including breast cancer and lung cancer, and chlorambucil, which is used for some lymphomas and some types of leukaemia.

The alkylating agents work by forming bonds between the two DNA strands, so that when they try to separate at the time of mitosis they are broken up.

The antimetabolites

These were the second group of anticancer drugs to be developed and first began to appear in the late 1940s. Two of the oldest drugs, still in general use today, are methotrexate and fluorouracil. Both of these are used to treat breast cancer. Fluorouracil is also used to treat cancer of the colon and rectum (large bowel cancer), and methotrexate is also used to treat cancer arising in the head and neck area. These days fluorouracil is usually given together with a vitamin called leucovorin, which increases its effectiveness.

More recent antimetabolites include gemcitabine (Gemzar), useful for cancer of the pancreas; fludarabine (Fludara), for use against some lymphomas; capecitabine (Xeloda), for large bowel cancer; and pemetrexed (Alimta) for the asbestos-related cancer mesothelioma.

The antimetabolites all work by interfering with the production of new DNA, so that the cells are unable to make the material they need to produce new genes.

The anthracyclines

These are one group of a number of cytotoxic drugs that were developed from antibiotics. The two most important agents are epirubicin and doxorubicin. They are used in the treatment of breast cancer, lung cancer, stomach cancer and some lymphomas.

They act by inserting themselves between the DNA strands, fitting rather like a key in a lock, and so wedging the strands together such that they cannot separate at the time of mitosis.

Other cytotoxic drugs derived from antibiotics include bleomycin, which is used to treat testicular cancer, and mitomycin, which is given for stomach cancer.

Platinum compounds

These are all based on the heavy metal platinum. They were discovered by accident in the late 1960s, when studies looking at the effect of electric currents on the growth of bacteria found that if probes made of platinum were used to supply the current the bacteria died off. Further studies showed that, rather like the alkylating agents, platinum compounds can produce crosslinks between the DNA strands, stopping the reproduction process.

The three platinum compounds in common use today are cisplatin and carboplatin (Paraplatin), which are valuable in ovarian cancer, lung cancer and testicular tumours, and more recently oxaliplatin (Eloxatin), which is used against cancers of the colon and rectum (bowel cancers).

Spindle poisons

These are drugs that interfere with a substance called tubulin, which is present in the cells. One of the things that tubulin does is to make the cell spindle, which separates the new chromosomes during mitosis. So the damage to tubulin prevents the cell spindle from working properly and arrests the process of cell division.

The spindle cell poisons are all based on natural compounds. One group are the vinca alkaloids, from the periwinkle plant *Vinca rosea*. These include vincristine (Oncovin) and vinblastine (Velbe), which are valuable in lymphoma treatment, and vinorelbine (Navelbine), which is used to treat breast and lung cancer. The second group are the taxanes, based on extracts from the bark of the Pacific yew tree. These are paclitaxel (Taxol) and docetaxol (Taxotere). They are used mainly against breast and lung cancer.

Topoisomerase inhibitors

Topoisomerases are a group of enzymes that help with the reproduction of DNA in the nucleus. Topoisomerase inhibitors damage the enzymes and stop new DNA formation.

These drugs include etoposide (Etopophos, Vepesid), which is used in lung cancer and testicular cancer; irinotecan (Campto), which is used to treat large bowel cancer; and topetecan (Hycamtin), which is used to treat ovarian cancer.

Combination cytotoxic chemotherapy

Occasionally a single cytotoxic drug will be given, but usually a combination of drugs is used. These combinations are made up of several drugs that work in a variety of different ways to interfere with cell division in order to maximize the effectiveness of the treatment.

There are countless different combinations of drugs used for the numerous different types of cancer, and new regimens are being devised and tested all the time. They are often known by acronyms, based on the names of the drugs that are given. For example, one of the most widely used treatments for testicular cancer is BEP, which is a combination of the drugs bleomycin, etoposide and cisplatin. Similarly, a commonly used treatment for Hodgkin lymphoma is

ABVD, which includes Adriamycin, bleomycin, vinblastine and dacarbazine. Doctors often call these combinations 'chemotherapy regimens' or 'chemotherapy regimes'.

It is important to give a word of reassurance at this point. For some types of cancer the number of cytotoxic regimens available is very limited, but for others there are many different options. For example, in breast cancer, bowel cancer and lung cancer, clinical trials have shown that several different combinations of cytotoxic drugs are equally effective in treating the condition. But this can lead to confusion and anxiety when people know that they are having a particular cocktail of drugs for their cancer and then find that a friend or relative being treated at another hospital, for a similar type of cancer, is having a different cytotoxic regimen. Understandably, they wonder why different treatments are being given and are anxious that one treatment might be better than the other. But almost always the answer will be that there is a variety of drug regimens that all work equally well and that different specialists have chosen different treatments based on their personal experience and the particular needs of individual patients (e.g. choosing a treatment that avoids particular side effects that someone might find especially upsetting, or a treatment that has a timetable that fits in well with their domestic arrangements). It is certainly not a case of one person getting a second-rate treatment, and neither will it be a case of someone getting a particular treatment because it is a cheaper option. Doctors will always choose the treatment that they think is best for each individual patient, irrespective of cost, provided that it is available on the National Health Service (see 'Costs and postcode prescribing', page 26).

Hormonal treatments

Hormones can play an important role in the treatment of a few types of cancer, most notably breast and prostate. This is because about six out of ten breast cancers and at least nine out of ten prostate cancers need a supply of hormone to encourage their growth. The breast cancers are dependant on the female hormone oestrogen, and the prostate cancers need the male hormone androgen. These sex hormones, which are normally present in the blood stream, bind to a special protein in the cancer cell called a receptor. Once the hormone has attached to the receptor, this sends signals to the nucleus of the cell encouraging it to divide.

Simple tests can be done to see whether a breast cancer contains oestrogen receptors (a tumour that does have receptors is known as 'ER-positive', one that doesn't is 'ER-negative', with the abbreviation 'ER' being based on the American spelling of 'estrogen'). Only an ER-positive breast cancer is likely to respond to hormone treatments; ER-negative cancers are usually unaffected by them. Prostate cancers are not routinely tested to look for androgen receptors because they are so common that is assumed that they will always be present.

Hormonal treatments are sometimes called endocrine therapies, because hormones are made by a group of glands known as the endocrine glands.

Hormonal, or endocrine, treatments work in one of two ways: by reducing the level of sex hormone – oestrogen or testosterone – in the blood stream (so the receptor is not stimulated); or by binding to the receptor, which stops the sex hormones attaching to it and activating the receptor.

In breast cancer the drugs given to lower the level of oestrogen in the blood stream depend on whether you have gone through the menopause. For women who are still having periods the drug goserelin (Zoladex) is used, whereas for women who are past the menopause one of a family of drugs called aromatase inhibitors may be given. These include anastrazole (Arimidex), exemestane (Aromasin) and letrozole (Femara). The most important drug for blocking the oestrogen receptor is tamoxifen, and this can be given to women of all ages. A newer drug that binds to and inactivates the receptor is called fulvestrant (Faslodex), and this agent is currently being assessed.

In prostate cancer either goserelin (Zoladex) or a similar drug such as leuprorelin (Prostap) or triptorelin (Decapeptyl, Gonapeptyl) can be used to lower the level of the male hormone testosterone in the blood stream. There are also a number of drugs that block the androgen receptors, and these include bicalutamide (Casodex), flutamide (Drogenil) and cyproterone acetate (Cyprostat).

Although hormonal treatments can be very important, they

are not usually given at the same time as cytotoxic chemotherapy because giving the two treatments simultaneously has been shown to reduce their effectiveness.

Targeted therapies

From the 1970s onward scientists have discovered a number of other receptor systems that are linked to cancer cells. These different receptors are either unique to cancer cells or are found in far greater numbers on cancer cells than in normal cells. The receptors lie on the outer surface of the cell, the cell membrane. They are made up of an outer part, projecting from the cell surface, and an inner part, projecting into the cytoplasm of the cell. Different growth factors circulating in the blood stream bind to the outer part, and when this happens chemical changes take place that stimulate the inner part of the receptor to send signals to the cell nucleus, telling it to start the process of mitosis or cell division. A key chemical in this process is an enzyme called tyrosine kinase, and so these different receptors are often known as tyrosine kinase receptors. The discovery of these receptors has led to new drugs being developed that can attack them, thereby stopping the growth of the cancer.

One of the limitations of cytotoxic drugs is that they cannot distinguish between cancer cells and normal cells, and so they interfere with cell division in both normal and cancerous tissues. This leads to unwanted side effects. Because the tyrosine kinase receptors are either unique to certain types of cancer cell or are found in far greater concentrations in cancer cells than in normal cells, drugs that attack them cause relatively little damage to normal cells and so have less severe side effects than cytotoxic drugs. Because they focus on cancer cells, these drugs have become known as targeted therapies.

Research into tyrosine kinase receptors and targeted therapies to inactivate them is a very exciting development in cancer treatment. So far relatively few drugs that work in this way have become available for routine treatment, but it is likely that we will see more and more of these agents appearing in the coming years and they will become increasingly important in cancer treatment.

The drugs that are currently available are of two main types. Drugs in one group are directed toward inactivating the external part of the tyrosine kinase receptor, stopping growth factors from attaching to it and stimulating it. These drugs are usually a type of compound called a monoclonal antibody. Examples of these monoclonal antibodies include rituximab (MabThera), which is used to treat some lymphomas; trastuzumab (Herceptin), which is used for some breast cancers; and bevacizimab (Avastin), which is being assessed in colorectal and other cancers. The other group of drugs are simple chemical compounds that attack the internal part of the receptor and stop it sending signals to the cell nucleus. These include imatinib (Glivec), which is used to treat a particular type of leukaemia (chronic myeloid leukaemia), sunitinib (Sutent) for kidney cancer and erlotinib (Tarceva) for some types of lung cancer.

The targeted therapies may be used on their own or they may be given alongside cytotoxic or hormonal treatments.

A note about steroids

The word 'steroids' is shorthand for a family of different hormones produced by the adrenal glands (two small glands that sit on top of each of our kidneys). One group of steroids are called corticosteroids, and two synthetic versions of these hormones, called prednisolone and dexamethasone, are often used in cancer treatment.

These steroids can be given for a number of different reasons. Sometimes they form part of an actual chemotherapy treatment schedule. Particularly in cancers like leukaemias and lymphomas, steroids boost the effectiveness of cytotoxic drugs and so are combined with them as part of the anti-cancer therapy. Dexamethasone is also quite effective in helping to prevent or reduce the sickness caused by chemotherapy. It is therefore often given along with other anti-sickness drugs at the time chemotherapy is being given and for a few days afterward.

In some types of cancer, especially brain tumours and some lung cancers, some of the symptoms are due to inflammation caused by the tumour in the tissues that surround it. Steroids help to reduce inflammation, and dexamethasone is particularly effective at doing this and so it is often given as part of the treatment for these tumours, leading to rapid improvement in troublesome symptoms like headache and breathlessness.

For people who have advanced, widespread cancer, steroids like prednisolone and dexamethasone can often be very effective tonics. They help to increase appetite, ease sickness, improve energy levels and make for a better quality of life with a general feeling of well-being.

Understandably, given all the publicity about various types of steroids, and their abuse by athletes and others, people often worry when their doctors tell them that they will be having steroids as part of their cancer treatment. In most cases, however, the drugs are only used for short periods of a few days or weeks at a time, and when they are given in this way side effects are uncommon.

A note about bisphosphonates

The bisphosphonates are a group of drugs that help to strengthen the bones. They are being increasingly used for people who have cancers that have spread to affect their bones. The three conditions in which they are being used most frequently are myeloma (a type of cancer that affects the marrow in the bones and leads to bone damage), breast cancer and prostate cancer.

People often confuse these drugs with chemotherapy because they are sometimes given as a drip into a vein in the arm once every few weeks (although they can sometimes be given as tablets). However, they are completely different from cytotoxic and other types of chemotherapy. They also usually have very little in the way of side effects.

Bisphosphonates can be given for a number of reasons. For people who have cancers that have spread to their bones, giving these drugs can help reduce the risk of complications such as fractures and abnormally high calcium levels in the blood (hypercalcaemia). Hypercalcaemia is a quite common, and sometimes serious, complication of bone secondaries. The high levels of calcium in the blood lead to symptoms of feeling thirsty, passing a lot of urine, feeling generally ill and sometimes becoming muddled and confused. Bisphosphonates can be used to prevent hypercalcaemia or to treat it if it develops. Sometimes, giving bisphoshponates can also be helpful in controlling pain from bone secondaries. Finally, clinical trials are also underway to see whether these drugs can prevent bone secondaries from developing in women with breast cancer who are thought to be at particularly high risk of getting bony spread of their disease.

The development of bisphosphonates is a very active field in medicine, and new drugs are being introduced all the time. Some of the most widely used are pamidronate (Aredia), clodronate (Bonefos), etidronate (Didronel), zoledronic acid (Zometa) and ibandronic acid (Bondronat).

Incidentally, bisphosphonates are used in a number of non-cancerous bone conditions, like some types of osteoporosis (bone thinning), and so the fact that someone is on one of these drugs does not necessarily mean that they have cancer.

Costs and postcode prescribing

Chemotherapy can be very expensive. Some of the older drugs, which have been available for the past 30 or 40 years, cost only a few pounds, but some of the newer drugs cost hundreds of pounds, and sometimes more than a thousand pounds, for a single dose. Also, in recent years increasing numbers of these new and expensive drugs have become available.

In England and Wales currently, when it has been demonstrated that a new drug is effective and safe for the treatment of a particular condition, the authorities issue a product licence, which means that the drug can be marketed. Before a new cancer drug can be given on the NHS it must also be approved by the National Institute for Health and Clinical Excellence (NICE), which looks not only at the benefits and side effects of the drug but also at its cost-effectiveness. Only when NICE has given its approval can NHS doctors prescribe it (Scotland and Northern Ireland have similar but slightly different systems). This has caused problems because sometimes there can be a gap of months or even years between a product licence being issued and NICE giving its approval; in other instances NICE has not approved a drug even though a product licence has been issued. The latter situation means that someone who is being treated in a private clinic could get access to the drug, but someone else who is receiving treatment on the NHS would not be able to have it.

For people who feel that they need a particular drug that does have a product licence but has not been approved by NICE, there are two options. One is that they can buy the drug themselves and ask their NHS hospital team to give it to them (the NHS altered its rules during 2008 to allow this to happen), but this could still mean having to find thousands of pounds every month to cover the cost of the drug. The alternative is for the individual patient to make a 'special case' to their local primary care trust (PCT) asking them to fund the treatment. There is good evidence that the chances of success with this approach vary enormously across the country, with some PCTs agreeing to almost all requests and others agreeing to virtually none. This huge variation has led to the idea of a 'postcode lottery', with your chances of getting treatment paid for depending entirely on where you live.

At the present time (early 2009) the Department of Health is planning to introduce changes to NICE both to speed up the process for assessing new drugs and to alter the rules for deciding whether a drug is cost-effective, with the hope being that this will mean that more cancer drugs will become available more quickly. For the present, however, some people may find that the drug their doctor believes offers the best chance of success in their particular condition – even if it is available commercially – is not available on the NHS.

4

What is involved?

The chemotherapy that someone might need varies enormously, depending on the type of cancer they have and the stage of the disease (whether it is early or more advanced and widespread). At its simplest, treatment involves no more than taking a tablet once a day; at its most complex it may mean many months of intensive treatment as an inpatient on the ward. However, these are extremes, and for most people treatment will mean a number of visits as an outpatient or day-patient at a chemotherapy unit over a period of about six months. These chemotherapy units are run by specially trained staff and are only available at certain hospitals. This may mean that your local hospital will not be able to give you the treatment, and you may have to travel some distance to get to your nearest chemotherapy unit.

Who gives the treatment?

Cancer chemotherapy is a very specialized area of medicine. Therefore, although your initial care may have been under a surgeon or physician, they will usually refer you to another of their consultant colleagues if you need cytotoxic treatment. Most chemotherapy is given either by a medical oncologist (who specializes exclusively in drug treatment of cancer) or by a clinical oncologist (a consultant who is qualified to give both chemotherapy and radiotherapy). If you have a leukaemia, lymphoma or myeloma, your chemotherapy is likely to be given by a consultant called a clinical haematologist.

The consultant will decide what treatment you need, and be responsible for your overall care while you are receiving that treatment. However, your chemotherapy will usually be given by specialist chemotherapy nurses, and they will look after many of your day to day needs and problems throughout the treatment.

Starting off

When you first meet the specialist who will look after you during your chemotherapy, they will usually start by going through your medical history and the details of your present problem. They will probably also want to do a physical examination and check the results of any tests, such as scans or x-rays, that you have had.

They will then discuss your treatment with you. They may make a clear-cut recommendation, based on what they think is best for you, or it may be that there are different options for treatment and that – when these have been explained – you can actually choose which you would prefer. Usually, if there is a choice involved you would be given time to make a decision and wouldn't be expected to make up your mind there and then.

In outlining your treatment, the doctor should explain why you need it, what the aim is (whether the hope is to cure the cancer or to control it for some time, increasing life expectancy, or to relieve distressing symptoms) and what is involved. The latter may include how the treatment will be given (tablets, injections or drips), whether it will mean a stay in hospital at any time, how often it needs to be done, how long it will go on for and what side effects you might experience.

This first visit is obviously very important, and it is a very good idea to have someone with you – a friend or relative – who can help you to remember what was said and compare notes with you after-ward. Although you will usually be given some written information at the time, it still helps to have someone there who can talk things through with you at home. It is also worthwhile to make a list of questions that you want to ask about your cancer and its treatment before you see your specialist. It is likely that they will answer most of your queries as they are explaining things to you, but you can use your list to check on this and as a prompt to make sure that all your questions are answered. Having things written down is a wise precaution because, however carefully you prepare, your mind can often go blank during a consultation.

In its Cancer Reform Strategy document published at the end of 2007, the Department of Health outlined plans to introduce bespoke information prescriptions. These would give every patient a written record of all the information they had been given at each stage of their cancer journey. At the present time, mid-2009, pilot schemes are looking at how these can be brought into routine oncology clinics.

Once you have agreed on the proposed treatment with your specialist, they will usually ask you to sign a consent form. This confirms that you feel everything has been properly explained to you and that you are willing to go ahead with the chemotherapy.

The doctor will then arrange the date for your first treatment, but you may need some routine blood or other tests before this can be confirmed. Depending on the drugs you are going to be given, these tests may be done to check various things including your blood count, kidney function and liver function, and to ensure that your heart is working well. The doctor will probably also measure your height and weight, because these are used to work out the actual doses of some of the drugs that you may be given.

The chemotherapy nurses

Before you actually start your chemotherapy, you may well have a visit arranged to see the chemotherapy unit and meet the specialist nurses who will be looking after you during your treatment.

This preliminary visit can be useful in a number of ways. It obviously gives you the chance to see where you will have your treatment, get a feel for what is likely to be involved and meet the people who will be giving you your treatment. But it also gives you the chance to ask any questions you have thought of since you saw your specialist.

At this visit you may well be given some more written information about your treatment. This will often include your own 'handheld record'. This is a booklet that includes details about the chemotherapy unit, including contact telephone numbers for use if you have problems in between your visits. It usually also has a diary section where you can record your own details of the treatment, your blood test results and any other notes.

Having chemotherapy

Sometimes chemotherapy involves no more than taking tablets on a regular basis, but often it means having drugs given directly into a vein. This may involve having injections over a matter of a few minutes or having an infusion (a drip) over an hour or so, or a continuous infusion, where the drug is given through a pump over days or weeks. Nowadays, if you are going to have a lot of injections and blood tests you may be offered a venous line to make this easier for you (see page 32).

Usually, you will receive chemotherapy as an outpatient. The pattern of your visits will vary with the type of chemotherapy. If you are having cytotoxic drugs, these are usually given on a single day, or over a few days in succession followed by a gap of between two and four weeks before the next course. This interval is to allow normal cells to recover from the side effects of treatment before the next course is given. (Cancer cells recover much more slowly from the damage caused by cytotoxic drugs. Therefore, the spacing out of treatment into a number of courses, or cycles, means that in the long term there should be relatively little injury to normal cells but the cancer cells will have been destroyed.)

Before each course of treatment you will normally have a blood test. This checks your blood count, looking at your haemoglobin level (whether you are anaemic), the number of white blood cells (which prevent you getting infections) and the number of platelets (if these drop too low you are at risk of getting abnormal bleeding). All of these can be affected by cytotoxic chemotherapy, so it is important to make sure their levels are safe before the drugs are given.

With some treatments, you will need to take some tablets or medicines a few hours before each session, as a 'pre-med', to prevent or reduce side effects. You will usually also have drugs given – either into the vein or as tablets – at the time your cytotoxic chemotherapy is given, which will also help to prevent any unpleasant after effects. You are also likely to receive a supply of tablets to take at home during the few days after treatment, to stop any nausea or vomiting.

If you are having hormonal treatment or one of the newer targeted drugs, these generally cause fewer and less severe side effects than the cytotoxic agents. This means that they are usually given continuously, with no need for rest intervals and recovery periods. If you are having the drugs in tablet form, they will often be given on a daily basis; if they are being given intravenously, as a drip, then this might be once weekly or once a fortnight. Some hormone preparations are also given as injections under the skin (subcutaneous injections), and these may be given every month or once every three months.

Also with hormonal and targeted treatments, you will usually not need so many regular tests during your course of treatment. But you will, of course, have regular check ups with your clinical team to make sure that everything is going according to plan.

Overall, your treatment may continue anywhere from a few weeks to many years. Most cytotoxic treatment is completed within five or six months, but hormonal treatments may go on for five to ten years and some of the targeted therapies may need to be taken for the rest of your life.

Venous lines

Having a course of chemotherapy may involve a lot of needles, both for all the blood tests that need to be done and to give you the drugs themselves. Having a venous line offers an alternative to this. The line is a fine hollow silicone rubber tube, or catheter, which is inserted into a vein and stays in place throughout the time of your course of chemotherapy. Two types of line are used: a central line or a peripherally inserted central catheter (PICC) line.

The central line is inserted through the skin just below your collar bone into a large vein called the subclavian vein, and it is threaded along this until its tip lies in another large vein, namely the superior vena cava, just above your heart. Central lines are also sometimes known by the names of the manufacturers of the lines, the two main ones being Hickman and Groshong.

A PICC line (also known as a peripheral line) is inserted through one of the large veins near the bend of your elbow, and threaded along this through the subclavian vein and into the superior vena cava. Once in place, the line can be used to take blood for any tests you need during your treatment and to give you all the drugs that would normally have to be injected into a vein or given through a drip. The line is usually quite comfortable and can stay in place for a year or more if necessary.

Putting in the line is quite a simple procedure. You can have a PICC line placed as an outpatient, and the procedure does not need a general anaesthetic. The skin where the line is to be inserted is numbed with some local anaesthetic, and threading the line through the veins is usually quite painless, so you shouldn't have much discomfort when this is being done. The insertion only takes a few minutes, and you will have a chest x-ray immediately afterward to make sure that the tip of the line is in the right place. Putting a central line in is very similar, but sometimes this may be done with a short general anaesthetic rather than a local anaesthetic.

Once the line is in place it is important that it doesn't get blocked. To prevent this it will have to be flushed through with special fluid once or twice a week. Your nurses may ask you to come to the hospital to have this done, or they may arrange for a nurse to visit you at home. Sometimes it may be possible for them to teach you, or a friend or relative, how to flush the line.

Normally, lines are trouble free. The commonest problems that do occur are infections and blockages from small blood clots. Your chemotherapy nurses will always know what to do if you do have any difficulties with your line.

Venous lines can be very helpful for people who need a lot of injections, blood tests and drips during their treatment; they are also valuable for people who can't bear the thought of needles and for people who have 'poor' veins that are problematic for getting blood or injecting fluids. Lines are also essential for people who are having their chemotherapy continuously, through a pump, over a period of days or weeks.

It is simple to remove the line, and the procedure is done in the outpatient clinic, with just a local anaesthetic to avoid any discomfort; it only takes a few minutes.

Although the idea of having a line that stays in place for some months may seem a little strange, once it is in place it is usually trouble free. People soon get used to them and find that they really don't interfere with everyday life.

Implantable ports

These are a variation on venous lines. The line is placed in a similar way but instead of coming out on the skin it ends in a subcutaneous port. This is a small soft plastic bubble, about 2.5 to 4 centimetres (1 to 1.5 inches) across, which lies just under the surface of the skin. This means it is less obvious than a central or a PICC line, and it appears as just a little bump under the skin. It is usually placed near the top of the front of the chest.

Like central lines, implantable ports may be inserted either in the outpatient clinic, with a local anaesthetic, or occasionally as a day-patient procedure, if a general anaesthetic is used. They also need regular flushing to prevent them from becoming blocked.

Implantable ports (which are also known as portocaths) can be used just like the venous lines – to take blood tests or to give chemotherapy, blood transfusions or other intravenous fluids.

Infusion pumps

When a chemotherapy drug is given into a vein it is usual to set up a drip, with a bag of fluid on a drip stand, which trickles through a tube into the vein. The drug may either be given as an injection into the tubing of the drip, or it may be mixed with the fluid in the bag and run in as an infusion. Depending on the treatment that is being given, the drip may last for anywhere from a few minutes to a few hours.

But some chemotherapy treatments require the drugs to be given into a vein over a matter of days or even weeks. For these long infusions, a portable pump can be used along with a venous line. The pump is a battery driven device that holds a syringe, containing the chemotherapy drug. This is attached to the end of the venous line, and very slowly the pump squeezes a trickle of the drug into the vein. Once the infusion is complete, the pump is very simply disconnected.

Pumps vary in size but are usually little bigger than a mobile phone. They can worn in a special 'holster', which means they are easy to carry around and not very obvious. In this way treatment can continue when you are at home, and there should be very little effect on your normal day to day activities while the infusion is in progress.

Lumbar puncture

Very occasionally, most often with certain types of leukaemia, it may be necessary to give chemotherapy drugs into the space around the spinal cord – the major nerve that runs through the bones of the back (the vertebrae). This is so that the drug can reach parts of the nervous system that it might not get to if it were given by an ordinary infusion into a vein. This is known as epidural chemotherapy

This involves having a lumbar puncture, which can be done as an outpatient or a day-patient procedure. It involves having an injection of local anaesthetic into the skin over the lower part of your spine. Once the area is numb a needle is then slipped in between the vertebrae, into the spinal canal. Once the needle is in place the drug is injected over a few minutes. The needle is then removed. Usually, you will be asked to lie still, on your back, for an hour or so after the procedure before you go home. You may have a mild headache for up to 24 hours after the lumbar puncture.

5

What are the side effects?

In this chapter we will look at some of the main side effects of chemotherapy, and in the next chapter we will talk about how these can be prevented or reduced.

When someone first hears that they need chemotherapy, their biggest worry is usually the side effects of the treatment. Chemotherapy has a reputation for causing severe distress and disruption. While this can occasionally be true, it is important to make a few general points about the impact of chemotherapy, before we go into more detail about side effects.

Chemotherapy is not a single type of treatment. What is actually involved in having chemotherapy varies enormously and depends on the type of cancer you have and the stage it has reached. At one extreme, chemotherapy may be no more than taking a tablet once a day, with virtually no side effects at all; at the other end of the spectrum it may involve a year or more of intensive treatment, with long stays in hospital and possibly severe, even dangerous, complications. For most people, however, treatment will mean a number of visits to the chemotherapy unit, as an outpatient or a day-patient, over four to six months, with the possibility of some temporarily troublesome, but not very upsetting, side effects.

Different people react differently to the same treatment. Two people can be having an identical type of chemotherapy, for exactly the same type of cancer, and be of similar age with a similar level of general fitness, but whereas one will sail through treatment with virtually no problems, the other may experience a number of side effects, and their treatment may be quite a struggle.

This means that hearing about how other people have coped with their chemotherapy isn't necessarily a good guide to what will happen to you. First, they will probably have had a completely different type of treatment. Second, even if they have had similar drugs to you, their experience of the treatment may well be completely different to yours.

Certainly, before you start your treatment, your oncologist and the nurses who will be giving you your chemotherapy should have explained to you all of the common side effects that might occur with that treatment, and have given you an idea of how likely those side effects are and how troublesome they might be. They should also reassure you that they will give you help and support to deal with any problems that do occur, and give you contact telephone numbers so that you can get in touch with them at any time if unexpected problems develop. So, although no one will be able to predict in advance exactly how you will react to the treatment, you will have some idea of the sort of things that could happen, and know that there will be sympathetic nurses and doctors – with expert knowledge – who will help you cope if you do run into difficulties.

Most of this chapter will focus on the side effects of cytotoxic drugs, because most chemotherapy treatments still rely on the use of these drugs. Furthermore, it is these drugs that often cause troublesome, and sometimes serious, side effects. However, the problems associated with hormonal treatments and the targeted therapies will also be briefly discussed.

Common side effects of cytotoxic treatment

There are many different cytotoxic drugs, and many different combinations of these drugs are used in cancer treatment. This means that the likely side effects vary considerably depending on the drugs that are needed and the doses that are used. Having said this, there are some side effects that occur much more often than others. These include changes to your blood count (bone marrow suppression), sickness (nausea and vomiting), tiredness, hair loss (alopecia), mouth soreness and ulceration, and reduced fertility.

Changes to the blood count

Our blood contains three essential types of cell:

- the red blood cells (red corpuscles), which carry oxygen to the tissues;
- the white blood cells (white corpuscles), which help to protect us against infections; and
- the platelets, which prevent bleeding.

All of these cells are made by stem cells in the bone marrow, the spongy material that is inside many of the bones in our bodies. These stem cells are very sensitive to cytotoxic drugs and will often be damaged by them, which leads to fewer blood cells being produced.

If your stem cells are making fewer red blood cells than normal, this causes anaemia, making you tired and sometimes causing other symptoms, such as breathlessness. If too few white cells are being made you usually don't feel any different, but it does mean that your resistance is low and you are more likely to pick up infections. If too few platelets are produced then you are at greater risk of bruising easily and having abnormal bleeding.

Normally, the effect of a dose of cytotoxic drugs on the bone marrow cells is temporary. The changes come on a few days after treatment, reaching a peak at about 10–14 days and then recovering over the next week or so.

A simple blood test – the full blood count – gives a quick and accurate measurement of all of the different cells in the blood.

The production of white blood cells is the most sensitive to cytotoxic damage. If a blood count is done one or two weeks after a dose of chemotherapy, it will usually show a fall in the number of white blood cells. Changes to the red cells and platelets generally occur more slowly, and they are only likely to show up after several courses of the drugs (and very often are not affected at all during treatment).

When you are having cytotoxic chemotherapy you will have a full blood count before you start treatment, to make sure that your bone marrow is working properly and that all your blood cells are at a normal level. The blood count will then be repeated before each new course, or dose, of chemotherapy during treatment, to make sure that your cell counts have recovered and are at a safe level before the next treatment is given.

If the blood count has not recovered sufficiently, then the next treatment may be delayed or the dose of the drugs may be reduced, so that they do not damage the bone marrow cells any further.

Nausea and vomiting

Many cytotoxic treatments can make people feel sick. Very often this is bad enough to make them vomit. The feeling of sickness comes on a few hours after having the drugs. It is usually at its worst during the first two days after the chemotherapy has been given, and then it settles quite quickly over another day or two.

The risk of sickness, and its severity, varies enormously with different drugs. Some cause virtually no upset, whereas others can lead to very unpleasant sickness.

During the 1990s the prevention and treatment of nausea and vomiting caused by cytotoxic drugs improved quite dramatically. This was the result of new anti-sickness drugs that were introduced, which proved far more effective than older treatments.

It is important to realize that this change has taken place. Many people still remember friends or relatives who had their chemotherapy during the 1970s or 1980s and suffered very badly from sickness and vomiting, but nowadays this sort of problem is really very uncommon. You may feel a little bit queasy and a bit off your food for a day or so after each treatment, but this is usually the worst that you are likely to experience.

Tiredness (fatigue)

For many people tiredness is the main problem that they experience as a result of their cancer. This tiredness can have many causes – just having a cancer can often make you feel very weary. But there is no doubt that chemotherapy can also lead to tiredness.

The tiredness, or fatigue, due to cytotoxic chemotherapy usually comes on during the first week or two of treatment, and it often gradually gets more apparent as the course of treatment continues. Once the chemotherapy is over the sense of fatigue slowly reduces, but it can take anywhere from a month or two to more than a year before it completely disappears.

The tiredness is more likely if you are having, or have recently had, other treatments such as surgery or radiotherapy.

The feeling of fatigue can be very difficult to cope with. It can make even the slightest effort seem like a major task. Not only is there often a complete lack of energy, but the tiredness can also interfere with other things like your memory, your sleeping pattern and your sex life. It may also lead to symptoms such as breathlessness and loss of appetite. It can be difficult to feel interested in anything, and you often feel quite low and depressed.

Because it is not something that is easily measurable, like a change in your blood count, or not very obvious, like sickness and vomiting, fatigue has tended to be overlooked as a side effect of treatment in the past. But nowadays doctors and nurses are aware that it can be a big problem for many people, and there is often a lot that can be done to help. So, if your treatment does make you feel very tired, do let your medical and nursing team know this.

Hair loss (alopecia)

For many people the idea of having chemotherapy means that you must lose your hair. In fact, the risk of hair loss is linked directly to which drugs you are given. With some cytotoxic drugs hair loss almost always happens, whereas with others it is virtually unknown.

Your doctors and nurses should be able to let you know how likely alopecia (hair loss) is with your particular treatment, and what can be done to reduce the risk or cope with the problem when it develops.

When hair loss occurs, it usually develops about three to four weeks after starting treatment. Sometimes, once it starts it can progress very rapidly, with almost complete hair loss within a day or two; with other types of treatment it may be more a case of gradual thinning of the hair over several months.

Scalp hair is the most sensitive to the effects of chemotherapy, because it grows more rapidly than hair on other parts of the body. But sometimes the drugs will cause loss of eyebrows, eyelashes, underarm hair and pubic hair as well.

It is important to remember that however much hair you lose during your treatment, it will grow back again afterward (indeed, sometimes it even starts to grow while you are still having the drugs). Normally, the hair begins to reappear a month or so after the end of chemotherapy, and is back completely within three to six months. Often, however, it comes back with a different colour and appearance – a grey/black, 'pepper and salt' colouring, with quite a thick texture, and a slightly curly or wavy look is very common.

Sore mouth

Getting a sore mouth during cytotoxic chemotherapy is quite common. When this happens it usually comes on a few days after the drugs are given and settles within about a week.

If it does happen, the soreness can vary considerably in its severity. It is often no more than a slight discomfort, but sometimes it can be very uncomfortable and mouth ulcers can develop. Because your white blood cell count may be low at this time, the soreness may be aggravated by the development of fungal infections in the mouth – a condition known as oral thrush or oral monilia. This leads to whitish patches on the tongue and the lining of the mouth.

When mouth soreness develops it can also affect your sense of taste, so that things taste different or you may find you cannot taste things so well.

Reduced fertility

As with other side effects, the risk of any effect on fertility is related to which drugs are used, the doses given and the length of time the treatment goes on for. Some cytotoxic treatments carry a very high risk of infertility, but with others there is almost no risk.

For women, the likelihood of becoming infertile also relates to their age. The cytotoxic drugs that cause infertility do so by stopping the ovaries from making the female hormones that regulate the menstrual cycle. This leads to an early menopause, with periods stopping and often the onset of symptoms such as hot flushes, vaginal dryness and mood changes that are associated with the change of life. The risk of loss of ovarian activity with cytotoxic chemotherapy increases the closer a woman is to the natural menopause, so if you are a woman in your early twenties then your chances of infertility with a particular type of treatment will be less than for a woman in her mid-forties.

Sometimes cytotoxic chemotherapy leads to a temporary loss of ovarian activity, so the periods stop during treatment and for anywhere from three to 18 months afterward, but then can start again.

For men the risk relates almost entirely to which drugs are used. But in some types of cancer, in particular cancer of the testicle, a reduced level of fertility – with a lower than normal sperm count – may actually be part of their condition even before they start any treatment.

Because of the unpredictability of the effects of some types of cytotoxic chemotherapy on fertility, it would be wrong to think that having treatment acts as a reliable form of contraception. If you are practising birth control, then you should certainly continue this while you are having your chemotherapy.

More specific side effects of cytotoxic drugs

There are a number of side effects of cytotoxic drugs that, although important and occasionally serious, are limited to just a handful of the more commonly used agents. These include nerve damage, damage to the heart and lungs, kidney damage, allergic reactions, and skin and eye complications.

Nerve damage

When this happens it usually takes the form of a peripheral neuropathy. This affects the nerves in the arms and legs, usually beginning in the hands and feet. The first symptom is tingling, or pins and needles, in the fingers or toes. This gradually spreads to the rest of the hands and feet, and – if nothing is done – will go on to affect the rest of the limbs. As the condition progresses numbness of the affected areas will develop, and this leads to some loss of coordination, making fine movements – such as undoing buttons or tying shoelaces – more difficult. In its more advanced stages there may be weakness of the muscles in the arms and legs.

Peripheral neuropathy is a recognized complication of treatment with three groups of chemotherapy drugs: the vinca alkaloids (which include vincristine, vinblastine, vindesine and vinorelbine), the platinum compounds (cisplatin, carboplatin and oxaliplatin) and the taxanes (paclitaxel and docetaxel).

Another type of nerve damage, which is limited to the platinum drugs, especially cisplatin, leads to problems with hearing. This begins as noises in the ear – whistling, buzzing or ringing sounds (which doctors call tinnitus). This can lead on to an actual loss of hearing and deafness.

Both peripheral neuropathy and hearing problems (ototoxicity) only come on very gradually, over weeks or months, and are related to the doses of the drugs that are being given. Doctors are very well aware of these side effects and will regularly ask whether you are noticing any numbness, pins and needles, or have any ringing or buzzing in your ears if you are being given these compounds. If you do notice any of these symptoms, then do let your medical team know – they will be able to adjust your treatment before any harm is done.

Damage to the heart

A group of drugs called anthracyclines, which include doxorubicin and epirubicin, can cause damage to the heart muscle. This can lead to weakness of the heart muscle and heart failure. This only occurs after quite large amounts of the drug have been given over many months, and nowadays most of the dose schedules using these drugs ensure that the total amount of the drug given throughout the course of treatment is well within the safe level, where heart damage is extremely unlikely. It is usual, however, for people who are going to be given one of these drugs to have a routine heart test and ECG – or electrocardiogram – just to make sure their heart is quite healthy before they start treatment.

The group of drugs called taxanes (paclitaxel and docetaxel) can also affect the heart. They can interfere with the control of heart rhythm, leading to an irregular heart beat. Usually, even if this happens it does not cause any real symptoms or problems. The taxanes, especially docetaxel, can also lead to fluid retention, which shows itself by causing swelling of the ankles and lower legs (ankle oedema). Although ankle oedema is one sign of heart failure, the fluid retention caused by taxanes does not seem to be directly related to any effect on the heart.

One of the newer targeted therapies, trastuzumab (Herceptin), is also linked to heart damage and this will be discussed later (see 'Targeted therapies', page 48).

Lung damage

This is very uncommon, but two drugs – bleomycin and busulfan – when given at high doses can cause thickening of the tissues in the lung (lung fibrosis), which can lead to shortness of breath. Because this effect has been recognized, the doses of the drugs given are usually well below the levels at which this complication might develop.

Kidney damage

The platinum compounds, in particular cisplatin, can damage the kidneys, leading to partial kidney failure. Because of this, before someone has treatment with a platinum drug it is normal for him or her to undergo tests to check how well the kidneys are working. When this has been done, the drug can be prescribed at a safe level to ensure that the risk of any injury to the kidneys is minimal. Usually, simple blood tests, and sometimes more complex tests of renal (kidney) function, will be done during the course of treatment, before each dose of the drug, to make sure that there is no evidence of kidney damage developing.

With some other drugs, where removal of the chemical from the body by the kidneys is very important, tests of renal function may be done before treatment starts to ensure that the kidneys can handle the drug, even though the drug itself does not cause any damage to the kidney.

Allergic reactions

Some drugs, including the taxanes (paclitaxel and docetaxel) and bleomycin, may cause allergic or hypersensitivity reactions. These show up as fevers, or shivers and shakes, often with a feeling of weakness or sickness, which come on within a few minutes to an hour or so after starting the drug. Usually, this problem can be avoided by giving other drugs before the chemotherapy, which will prevent an allergic reaction from occurring.

Skin damage

Most chemotherapy drugs are given through a drip into a vein. Even when the drug is given very carefully, by trained skilled nurses, small amounts of the drug may occasionally leak outside the vein, into the surrounding soft tissues. This is called extravasation. With most drugs extravasation is not a problem and will only cause some very slight, brief discomfort at most. With a few drugs, however, any leakage into the tissues around the vein can cause quite severe inflammation, with redness, swelling and soreness. This comes on almost immediately after the extravasation has occurred and – depending on the drug and the amount that has leaked into the tissues – may take days or even weeks to settle down.

The drugs most likely to cause irritation and skin damage when they leak are anthracyclines (doxorubicin and epirubicin) and the vinca alkaloids (vincristine, vinblastine, vindesine and vinorelbine).

The risk of this kind of damage can be avoided by having a central line or peripherally inserted central catheter (PICC) line for your drug administration, but it is still a very uncommon problem – even if you are having your drugs through an ordinary drip into a vein in your arm. If it does occur, then putting ice packs on the area and having injections of steroids under the skin where the leakage has occurred will reduce the immediate discomfort and lessen the risk of any lasting skin damage or scarring. Using an anti-inflammatory cream on the affected area for a week or so afterward can also help.

A completely different type of skin damage can occur with the drugs fluorouracil and capecitabine. These can lead to a condition known as hand–foot syndrome. In hand–foot syndrome the skin of the palms of the hands and soles of the feet becomes red and sore, and may actually begin to blister and peel. It usually only comes on gradually, with higher doses of the drugs, and adjusting the dose will usually ease the problem. Sometimes, taking tablets of vitamin B_6, pyridoxine, can help and your doctor may prescribe these for you.

Eye complications

Serious eye problems are very rare indeed with cytotoxic drugs, but some drugs – in particular fluorouracil – can lead to a feeling of soreness or grittiness, with watering of the eyes. Soothing eye drops will usually ease this symptom.

Diarrhoea and constipation

A few drugs, in particular irinotecan and cisplatin, may cause diarrhoea, and occasionally this can be severe. If this is likely to happen your doctors and nurses will usually warn you about it and give you a supply of tablets or capsules that you can take if the problem develops. They will also advise you that drinking plenty of fluids, making sure that you don't get dehydrated, is important if you do get diarrhoea.

Constipation may occur if you are having vinca alkaloid drugs (vincristine, vinblastine, vinorelbine or vindesine). It is also a side effect of some of the drugs that are used to prevent sickness, and so you may find that you are a bit constipated during the first day or two after having your chemotherapy. Once again, drinking plenty of fluids helps to reduce the likelihood of a problem, and eating plenty of fresh fruit and fibre is a good idea.

Cancer formation

Over the 60 years that chemotherapy has been used, there have been occasional reports suggesting that giving cytotoxic drugs can actually lead to a risk of developing another cancer later in life. The likelihood of chemotherapy leading to cancer formation has been the subject of a very great deal of research. This has shown that although it is impossible to say that there is absolutely no risk, if there is a chance of cytotoxic chemotherapy drugs leading to cancer development then it is very, very small indeed, and that minute risk is far outweighed by the benefits of treatment.

Common side effects with hormonal treatments

Hormonal therapies are commonly used only in breast cancer and prostate cancer. Usually, they cause fewer and less serious side effects than cytotoxic chemotherapy, but they may still sometimes cause problems.

Side effects of hormonal therapies for breast cancer

Menopausal symptoms

Many women being treated for breast cancer have virtually no problems at all from their hormonal treatment. Having said this, for a small minority of women the therapy can be very upsetting. The most common problem is unpleasant menopausal side effects. These include hot flushes, drenching sweats, vaginal dryness and soreness, mood swings, feeling irritable and short tempered, loss of concentration and difficulty in remembering things.

About one in three younger women taking tamoxifen will find that their periods stop (if this happens it is still possible to become pregnant, and so it is important to continue contraception), one in three will find that their periods become irregular, and one-third will see no difference. However, all may get menopausal symptoms, as may some women who are postmenopausal and are given the drug.

With the drug goserelin (Zoladex) younger women will find that their periods stop completely. This is because the drug stops their ovaries from working, which also means that they become infertile. However, unlike many cytotoxic treatments, once the drug is stopped the ovaries will start working again and fertility will be restored and pregnancy will be possible (provided that the woman has not reached the age of her natural menopause).

Cancer of the womb

About one in every 500 women who take the drug tamoxifen for more than two years will develop cancer of the womb. This is because tamoxifen increases the growth of the cells that line the womb, and this may eventually lead to a cancer forming. If this happens it usually causes some bleeding from the vagina. So if you are taking tamoxifen and you ever develop any unexpected bleeding from your vagina then do let your doctors know as soon as possible so that they can check up on this for you. Happily, most womb cancers caused by tamoxifen therapy have been found at an early stage, and the cure rate has been very high.

Thrombosis

Another occasional side effect of tamoxifen is an increased risk of venous thrombosis – the formation of blood clots in the veins. The risk is quite small, with fewer than one in 100 women who take tamoxifen getting a thrombosis. But if you have a history of blood clots, do let your doctor know because it would probably be better if your treatment was changed to another type of hormonal therapy.

Osteoporosis (bone thinning)

The fall in the level of the female hormone oestrogen that happens when the ovaries stop working means that once you have passed the menopause you are more likely to develop thinning of the bones – osteoporosis. Taking one of the aromatase inhibitor drugs increases this risk. Exemestane (Aromasin), anastrozole (Arimidex) and letrozole (Femara) are the most widely used aromatase inhibitors. This is not the case with tamoxifen, which actually offers some protection against osteoporosis.

Side effects of hormonal therapies for prostate cancer

Most of the hormonal treatments used for prostate cancer may cause 'menopausal' hot flushes and sweats. Loss of interest in sex (reduced libido) and even impotence, with difficulty in getting an erection, may also be a problem, but this does not usually happen with bicalutamide (Casodex) and flutamide (Drogenil). However, about two-thirds of men who have one of these two drugs will have develop breast pain and sometimes some swelling and enlargement of their breast (which doctors call gynaecomastia), making their breasts more feminine in appearance.

Targeted therapies

The targeted therapies include a very diverse group of drugs, with a wide range of possible side effects. But compared with cytotoxic drugs, these side effects are generally much less serious and less upsetting.

One problem that has attracted a lot of publicity is the risk of heart failure caused by trastuzumab (Herceptin). This only occurs in a small number of people given this drug, but when it happens it causes weakening of the pumping of the heart, leading to shortness of breath and fluid overload (most often seen as swelling of the ankles). Although this sounds serious, the good news is that the heart failure normally responds very to well to treatment, and the problem disappears once trastuzumab is stopped.

A number of the targeted therapies have to be given by intravenous infusion (through a drip), and these can sometimes cause allergic reactions. These show up as shivering, fever and a skin rash that appears within a few minutes of starting the drip. Very occasionally a more severe type of reaction can occur (doctors call this cytokine release syndrome). This comes on an hour or so after the infusion has started and causes severe breathlessness and wheezing, as well as the skin rash, fever and shivering.

Skin rashes are also common with some targeted therapies, in particular the drugs cetuximab (Erbitux), erlotinib (Tarceva) and gefitinib (Iressa). These usually cause a rash that looks very much like acne. The rash usually fades after a few weeks, but it leaves the skin rather dry and liable to crack.

6

Coping with side effects

The previous chapter described many of the side effects that can occur with chemotherapy. Happily, for many people there will be relatively few problems during their treatment, but for others there may be troublesome and unpleasant symptoms. This chapter describes how to reduce the risk of the commoner problems and, when they do occur, how to cope with them and keep any upset to a minimum.

Infection

Nearly all cytotoxic drugs have an effect on the bone marrow, which leads to a reduction in the number of white cells circulating in the blood. Because the white blood cells are the body's main line of defence against infection, this means that you may be at greater risk of picking up an infection while you are having chemotherapy. As a rule, hormonal treatments and targeted therapies do not increase your risk of infection.

How badly the bone marrow is affected depends on the drugs that you are given and the doses that are used. Typically, the white cell count in the blood begins to fall about five to seven days after a dose of cytotoxics, and will reach its lowest level about two weeks after the treatment. After that the count recovers and will be more or less back to normal by the end of the third week. You will always have a blood test before the next dose of drugs is given; this is to make sure that your blood count has recovered sufficiently for it to be safe to carry on with the treatment.

Your doctors and nurses should warn you about the risk of infection while you are receiving treatment and explain how high that risk is in your particular case. The usual advice would be to let your hospital know immediately if, at any time during treatment, you get one or more of the following:

- a temperature above 38°C (>100.5°F);
- symptoms suggesting an infection, such as shivering, a sore throat, a cough and shortness of breath, or cystitis (stinging and burning when you pass urine and wanting to pass water more often than usual); and
- simply a sudden feeling of being unwell.

There will always be someone available to see you and advise what to do. Usually, they will talk to you, probably examine you and take a blood test. The hospital team should always give you contact telephone numbers so that you can get in touch at any time, night or day, and at weekends if you are worried. Do make sure that you have these and know where to find them if you need them.

If you do develop an infection, you can normally be treated for it as an outpatient with a course of antibiotics. But sometimes, for more severe infections or if your blood count is very low, you may need to go into hospital for a few days for intensive antibiotic therapy, with the drugs being given through a drip into a vein. You may also have injections of growth factors (granulocyte colony stimulating factors, or G-CSF), which are compounds that stimulate the bone marrow to produce more white blood cells and help to speed the recovery of the blood count. They are usually given as very small injections under the skin once or twice a day.

Occasionally, your time in hospital may involve something called reverse barrier nursing, where you are in a room on your own and when people come in they will have to wear gowns and masks, and either put on gloves or use special antibacterial hand washes. All this is done to protect you from picking up any further infections, and it is usually only necessary for a day or two until your white cell count begins to recover.

If you have had an infection after a dose of cytotoxic drugs, then your doctors may give you antibiotics to take before and during your remaining courses of treatment to prevent any further episodes. Less commonly, they may use injections of growth factors, G-CSF, during your remaining courses of treatment to try to boost your white blood cell levels.

Sometimes, if your medical team think that the drugs you'll be given will put you at high risk of picking up an infection, then they may start you on antibiotics before you begin your cytotoxic treatment, as a precaution to try to prevent this.

There are a number of things that you can do to help reduce your chances of getting an infection while you are having cytotoxic drugs. These include the following.

- Avoid friends or family members who have an obvious infection, such as a bad cold or flu, or children with illnesses such as measles, mumps or chicken pox. Chicken pox is particularly important because the virus that causes this is the same one that causes shingles (herpes zoster), and people who are having chemotherapy are particularly likely to get shingles.
- Avoid very crowded places where you will have to spend time close to large numbers of people, because you can never tell if any of them might be carrying an infection you could catch.
- Avoid swimming or other sports where you have to share changing rooms and showers with other people.
- Be very particular about your personal hygiene. Bath or shower at least once a day, and always wash your hands well after going to the toilet and before preparing any food or cooking. Try to make sure that you have your own flannel, towels and soaps, and don't share with other members of the family.
- Take care with oral hygiene too, because mouth infections are common with chemotherapy. Drink plenty of fluids (at least two litres, or four pints, each day) because this will keep your mouth moist and reduce the risk of an infection. Also brush your teeth at least twice a day, with a soft brush. Take advice from your doctors and nurses as to whether using a mouthwash as well might be a good idea.
- Drink plenty of fluids because this helps to reduce the chances of getting cystitis. There is also some evidence that having a glass of cranberry juice each morning and evening can help prevent urinary tract infection.
- If your doctors and nurses think you have a very high risk of getting an infection, or if your white blood count goes very low, then they may give you advice about what you should, or rather should not, be eating. This usually means avoiding raw foods such as salads, or foods that might naturally contain bacteria

such as cheeses and yoghurts. Takeaway foods are also not a good idea.

One thing people often ask about is whether they should have a flu jab. Having a flu jab won't do any harm but if your white cell count is very low, and your immunity is reduced, it may not be very effective and may not give you very much protection against getting influenza. The best thing, if you are going to have the jab, is to have it about two weeks before you first start your treatment. If you decide to have it after you have started cytotoxic treatment, then try to get it at a time when your white blood count is as near normal as possible (just before a course of treatment is due). Your nurses will be able to advise you of the best time and could arrange a blood test so that you can be sure your white cell level is reasonable. Having hormonal treatments or one of the targeted therapies usually won't affect your immunity, so it is fine to go ahead with the flu jab while you are taking these drugs.

Sickness: nausea and vomiting

Along with hair loss, sickness is the thing that most people fear about chemotherapy. Once again, this is most likely to be a problem during cytotoxic chemotherapy, but it can sometimes be troublesome with hormonal treatment or targeted therapies.

Until the early 1990s sickness was a major problem with cytotoxic drug treatment and could often be very difficult to control. However, the introduction of a new group of anti-sickness drugs (antiemetics) called the 5-hydroxytriptamine 3 (5HT3) antagonists brought about a huge improvement, so that nowadays severe sickness is something that very few people experience.

How likely you are to be sick and how bad that sickness will be depends on the drugs that are being given. Some cytotoxic drugs are much more likely to cause sickness than others. There is also evidence that some people are more vulnerable to cytotoxic drug-induced nausea and vomiting – women are more at risk than men, younger people are more at risk than older people, and a history of motion sickness means you are more likely to have problems.

The best way to manage chemotherapy-induced sickness is to prevent it from happening in the first place. This means that with any treatment in which nausea and vomiting are likely, you will be given antiemetics routinely before the cytotoxic drugs. Because most chemotherapy drugs are given through a drip into a vein, this usually involves having the antiemetics injected into the drip immediately before the cytotoxics. You will then usually have a supply of antiemetic tablets to take for a day or two afterward.

The effectiveness of antiemetics can be increased by giving a steroid drug, called dexamethasone, at the same time. People sometimes worry about 'having steroids' because of the risk of side effects, but because the drug is only given for a few doses during each course of treatment the risk of any problems is very small indeed.

Although the worst of any sickness from chemotherapy passes within a day or two, feelings of queasiness, and sometimes actually being sick, can persist for a week or even longer. These troublesome but less severe symptoms can often be controlled by milder antiemetics, which once again can be taken as tablets for up to a fortnight after treatment.

So, in a typical schedule for an antiemetic, you would receive a dose of a 5HT3 antagonist, such as ondansetron (Zofran) or granisetron (Kytril), along with a dose of dexamethasone given into a vein just before the chemotherapy is given. These would be followed by tablets of the 5HT3 antagonist and steroid to take regularly twice a day for the next two or three days. You would then have a supply of another type of antiemetic, typically metoclopramide (Maxolon) or domperidone (Motilium), to take as and when necessary to relieve any feeling of sickness over the next week or so. This schedule will prevent sickness altogether or keep it to a very low and tolerable level for the great majority of people. But everyone is different, and sometimes these measures will not be enough. If this is the case, then your doctors and nurses will be able to adjust the doses or timing of your anti-sickness drugs, or add in other antiemetics, to try to give you the maximum possible relief.

Although they are very effective at preventing and relieving sickness, some people do find that they get side effects from the 5HT3 antagonists. The commonest of these are constipation and headache. These can usually be relieved very easily, with a simple laxative such as Senokot, or a simple pain killer such as para-cetamol. If you do think you are getting side effects, then mention it to your chemotherapy nurses who will be able to advise you how to ease them.

A recent development is the introduction of a drug called aprepi-tant (Emend), which works in a different way to other anti-sickness drugs. It seems especially good at preventing the delayed sickness that may come on a day or two after treatment, which is a partic-ular feature of some drugs, especially one called cisplatin. It is given as a tablet, along with a 5HT3 antagonist and dexamethasone.

As well as taking the antiemetic medication you have been given by your chemotherapy team, there are a number of things you can try for yourself if you are feeling sick. These are included in the information box ('Coping with sickness').

Coping with sickness

- Avoid greasy, fatty or very spicy foods.
- Take ginger, since this helps to ease sickness, so try nibbling a ginger biscuit or drinking ginger ale or ginger beer.
- Avoid big meals, and eat little and often with light bites and snacks.
- If you feel sick first thing in the morning, keep a couple of dry biscuits by your bed and try to eat one before you get up.
- Make sure you have plenty of fresh air; keep a window open if you can, especially when cooking.
- If cooking smells upset you, try to get someone else to prepare your meals, or opt for cold food, with salads and sandwiches.
- Some people find that sea-bands can be helpful. These are bands that you strap round your wrists. They are fitted with a button that gently presses onto the skin over an acupressure point on the inner surface of the wrist. You can buy these sea-bands at any chemist.

Tiredness (fatigue)

Profound tiredness, or fatigue, is a very common problem during chemotherapy. It is thought that four out of five people having cytotoxics will experience fatigue on some days during their treatment, and for about one in three it will be present for most of the time. Even with hormonal treatment or targeted therapies tiredness can sometimes be a problem. Although it is something that affects many people, doctors have been slow to realize how important tiredness is as a side effect of cancer treatment, and they have concentrated on more obvious problems such as sickness and the risk of infection. This means there has been relatively little research into the causes and treatment of chemotherapy-related fatigue.

All of us get tired from time to time, but the fatigue that comes with chemotherapy can be much more severe than this. You may feel tired even when you are resting. Everyday activities – like washing yourself or making a cup of tea – can seem like major tasks. Concentrating on things is difficult, and meeting other people – even close friends and family – can be an ordeal.

An important thing to remember is that this tiredness is a very common feature of chemotherapy and it does not mean that the cancer is coming back or getting worse. Neither does it mean that things are going wrong with your treatment.

Although chemotherapy itself does cause weariness there can be other factors that might make the feeling worse. These include:

- anaemia, which is a common complication of cancer and its treatment;
- the presence of an infection;
- being clinically depressed; and
- being in pain.

All of these are things that can often readily be corrected. So if you are feeling very tired, then do mention it to your doctor and nurses so that they can check for these problems and arrange any treatment that may be necessary.

Many people don't tell their medical team when they feel worn out and lethargic, because they think that this is only to be expected and don't want to be a bother. But if you don't let them know then they won't be able to help you, so do speak up.

Anaemia can usually be rapidly reversed by a simple blood transfusion, which can often be given at the outpatient clinic. During the past year or two, doctors have discovered that even very mild levels of anaemia, which would not normally be troublesome, can lead to severe tiredness in people who are having chemotherapy, and correcting this can make a big difference to how they feel. Similarly, giving antibiotics or antifungal drugs for an infection, analgesics to relieve pain, or antidepressants to people who are clinically depressed can ease the feeling of tiredness quite dramatically.

But often fatigue is simply due to effects of chemotherapy, and when this is the case it is a matter of adjusting to cope with the situation. A few tips to help with this are provided in the information box ('Coping with fatigue').

Coping with fatigue

- Don't feel worried or, worse still, guilty. Severe tiredness during chemotherapy is quite natural, and it is something most people experience as part of their treatment. It is not your fault – it is the normal response of your body to all that is going on.
- Prioritize your activities. Do the things you have to do – like washing yourself or cleaning your teeth – but try to organize other people to do things like shopping or helping with the cooking.
- Plan your day. Keep a diary so you can see when you are likely to feel most tired (to help you plan rests) and see which things make you feel more tired (so you can avoid them). Try to plan as few trips up and down stairs as possible.
- Take regular rests or cat naps. If you feel you need to stop and put your feet up, then do so – don't push yourself to carry on.
- Make sure you sleep well at night. A warm bath and a hot milky drink at bedtime will often help, but if sleeping is a problem then let your doctors know and they may prescribe sleeping tablets to help.
- Avoid extremes of temperature. Getting over hot or feeling cold can be tiring.

- Eat healthily, including plenty of fresh fruit and vegetables, and drink at least two litres (four pints) of fluid every day.
- Find things to distract you and take your mind off the tiredness. Listening to pleasant music or relaxation tapes, watching daytime television and getting friends to take you out for a drive can all help (often activities that you would normally find trivial or boring can be much more entertaining and absorbing when you are tired).
- Try some gentle exercise. Although it may sound strange, there is good evidence that gentle exercise can often reduce fatigue. This not to say that you should sign up for the gym and attempt vigorous workouts, but – if you can manage it – a stroll round the neighbourhood for 20 to 30 minutes, five or six times a week, might make a big difference to how you feel.

Even when your course of chemotherapy is over, tiredness is likely to last for some time afterward, certainly for several months. Generally speaking, the older you are the longer it takes to recover your stamina, and if you have radiotherapy as well as chemotherapy then this can slow your return to normal energy levels. Studies suggest that even a year after treatment has finished, about one in five people will still regularly have days when they feel fatigued. So don't be worried if your lack of energy doesn't improve immediately, and allow for this in planning your life and activities after chemotherapy.

Mouth problems

These are most likely with cyotoxic chemotherapy. Cytotoxic drugs can affect your mouth in several ways. Sometimes they can cause a sore mouth. If this happens it usually comes on a few days after you have had your treatment. When you look in your mouth there may be nothing to see, or there may be some redness of the lining of your mouth (the mucosa) and sometimes there may be small ulcers. This inflammation and soreness of the lining of the mouth is called mucositis. If your blood count is on the low side, if you are on steroids or antibiotics, or if you are very run down, then you may also get an infection in your mouth. The most common type of infection is called thrush (also known as oral candidiasis or oral monilia). This usually shows up as small whitish patches on the mucosa and the surface of the tongue. Another quite common problem with cytotoxic treatment is getting a dry mouth, and this can also lead to changes of taste, with some foods and drinks tasting different from normal.

One drug that is particularly associated with oral mucositis is methotrexate. If this problem develops, then a short course of folinic acid (leucovorin) tablets for a day or two can help, and taking the tablets after subsequent courses of the drug greatly reduces the risk of any further mouth soreness.

A sore mouth

The chances of getting a sore mouth do vary depending on your treatment; some drugs or combinations of drugs are more likely to cause mucositis than others. Usually, your doctors or nurses will warn you if oral soreness is likely to happen, but if they don't mention it then you can always ask them about it. If it has been flagged up as a possible side effect, then there are a number of things you can do that will help to reduce the chances of it developing (see information box 'Preventing sore mouth').

Preventing sore mouth

- Have a routine check-up with your dentist before you start treatment, just to be sure that there are no obvious tooth or gum problems that need to be dealt with before your treatment.
- Suck crushed ice for 15–30 minutes before your chemotherapy is given, and continue this while you are having the drugs and for about half an hour afterward; this can sometimes prevent mouth soreness. Check with your chemotherapy nurses whether this might be a good idea in your case.
- Maintain good oral hygiene, which means cleaning your teeth at least twice a day. Using a normal toothbrush can be uncomfortable, so it may help to use a soft toothbrush or a child's brush. You may find that your usual toothpaste makes your mouth and gums sore, and changing to a brand for 'sensitive

teeth', such as Sensodyne Original or Macleans Sensitive, might help. Mouthwashes can also be useful, and you can try these if you find that brushing your teeth is really painful. There are preparations you can get from your chemist or supermarket that help prevent infection, including chlorhexidine, Corsodyl and thymol. For simply keeping your mouth clean you can make your own mouthwash with a teaspoon of baking powder (sodium bicarbonate) dissolved in a glass of warm water, and use this to rinse out your mouth thoroughly morning and night.

- Keeping your mouth moist is a good idea, and some tips for how to do this are given in the 'Dry mouth' section on page 61.
- Change your diet. There are some foods and drinks that can make your mouth sore if the mucosa is sensitive. These include very hot and spicy foods, vinegar, salt, neat spirits (whisky, brandy, gin, etc.) and acid drinks such as grapefruit juice and some types of orange juice. Avoiding these might be a good idea.

If you get a sore mouth then do mention it to your nurses or doctors. They will be able to check for signs of infection and give you advice on what to do. If you have thrush, then this is easily treated by a course of antifungal drug such as nystatin or amphotericin for a few days. These drugs are given as either a pastille to suck four times day, or as a mouthwash that you rinse round your mouth and then swallow, again four times a day. If there is no evidence of infection, then some of the other things you can do to help a sore mouth after your chemotherapy are given in the information box 'Coping with sore mouth'.

Coping with sore mouth

- Use a pain-killing mouthwash. Difflam oral rinse is a mouthwash that can help; you can buy it over the counter. It is also available as a spray. Some people find that using the full-strength mouthwash stings, and diluting it with an equal amount of warm water may help. An alternative is to make your own mouthwash using soluble aspirin, dissolving a couple of tablets in a glass of warm water, and using this to rinse your mouth well three or four times a day.

- If you have mouth ulcers then there is a wide range of gels, pastes and sprays that might help. These include Bonjela gel, Biora gel, Medijel and Rinstead contact pastilles, and many more. Your local pharmacist will always be able to advise you about what is on offer.
- Sometimes taking a mild painkiller can be helpful. Paracetamol capsules or soluble paracetamol tablets taken two or three times daily may reduce your discomfort.

Usually, the mucositis associated with chemotherapy only lasts a few days and will have disappeared completely within a week or so.

A dry mouth

If you get a dry mouth during your treatment there are a number of things that might help (see information box 'Coping with dry mouth').

Coping with dry mouth

- Keep your mouth moist with regular fluids. You should be drinking at least two litres (four pints) of fluid every day during your treatment, but supplementing this with regular sips of water or other soft drinks can help (fizzy water or fizzy drinks tend to be better than still fluids). Sucking ice cubes or crushed ice is another idea.
- Smearing the surface of your tongue and the lining of your mouth with a little olive oil or melted butter will keep things moist for a while and is often particularly effective last thing at night.
- Chewing sugar-free chewing gum or sugar-free fruit pastilles can help to stimulate your salivary glands to make moisture for your mouth. In the same way, sucking pineapple chunks might help.
- Cleaning your mouth regularly with baking powder (sodium bicarbonate) mouthwashes – one teaspoonful of powder in a glass of warm water – keeps the mucosa moist and clean.
- Drinking a glass of sherry (especially dry rather than medium or sweet sherry) about a quarter of an hour before a meal can often stimulate the salivary glands, and your digestive system, to make eating easier and more appealing.

- Moistening your food helps, using plenty of gravy or sauces. Dry foods are best avoided, especially things like crackers, flaky pastry and chocolate, which all tend to stick to the lining of your mouth.
- There are a number of over the counter preparations of artificial saliva that some people find useful. These may come as sprays, gels or pastilles, and include Saliva Orthana, Glandosane, Luborant, Saliveze and Salivix. Once again, your local pharmacist will be happy to advise you about what is available.
- Using a lip balm to moisten your lips and keep them soft might make a difference.
- There are also some things to try and avoid. Smoking, alcohol and caffeine (in tea and coffee) all tend to make your mouth dry, so cutting back on these is a good thing.

Hair loss

Hair loss is a major worry for many people when they are first told they need chemotherapy, but it is usually only a problem with cytotoxic treatment. The likelihood of losing your hair varies greatly with different cytotoxic treatments. With some drugs hair loss (alopecia) hardly ever happens, but with others it is almost inevitable. When there is alopecia it may be anything from some thinning of the hair of the head to complete loss of all body hair.

If your treatment does involve drugs that carry a high risk of alopecia, the one thing that can sometimes be done to try to prevent or reduce this is scalp cooling. There are various types of scalp cooling, but the general principle is to chill the scalp, usually by wearing a special padded hat that contains a gel. The hat is stored in a freezer and is then strapped firmly on your head about half an hour before you are due to have your drugs.

You carry on wearing the hat while the drugs are given and for about half an hour afterward. If your drugs are being given over more than a few minutes, you may need to have your hat changed to make sure that your scalp remains chilled.

The idea behind this is that keeping the scalp very cold makes the blood vessels in the skin of your head contract, so that the blood supply to the hair follicles is reduced and they will be less affected by the circulating chemotherapy drugs.

Scalp cooling doesn't always work. For many people it will prevent or greatly reduce the amount of hair loss, but for others it has very little effect. Some people find scalp cooling uncomfortable. The hat is very cold and can often cause headaches, so it does not suit everyone. Scalp cooling only helps to preserve the hair on your head, and it won't stop hair loss anywhere else.

If you do develop alopecia then your chemotherapy team will give you advice on ways to cope with this. The most obvious of these is having a wig. These can be supplied by the NHS. Most chemotherapy departments have a specially trained member of staff who can discuss the options with you and arrange for you to have a wig that meets the colour and style you would like. There is usually a cost for this – the standard NHS charge is about £50 – but some hospitals have special funds that allow them to be provided free of charge. Alternatives to wigs include headscarves and bandannas, which allow some people to turn their hair loss into a fashion statement!

A small bonus is that some men find that while they are having chemotherapy they don't need to shave.

It is important to remember that if you develop alopecia it will always be temporary. However much hair you lose, it will grow back again within a few months of completing your chemotherapy – although it does often come back with a different colour and texture, often being curly or wavy, with a 'pepper and salt' colouring and slightly thicker, coarser texture.

Fertility

Chemotherapy can affect fertility for both men and women. The risk of becoming infertile varies greatly with the different treatments. After some types of cytotoxic and hormonal therapy sterility is inevitable, whereas with targeted therapies it is usually not affected. Not all cytotoxic and hormonal treatments cause infertility; with some it always happens, but with others it is almost unknown. Also, some drugs may cause infertility that is only temporary, lasting anywhere from a few months to a year or so, whereas with others it is likely to be permanent. If you are having hormonal treatment and become infertile then this is usually reversible, and your fertility will return after the treatment is completed. So if you are thinking that you might want to have children in the future, do discuss this with your doctors before you start treatment so that they can work out the treatment that is least likely to interfere with your fertility while still being effective against the cancer.

If there is still a likelihood that treatment will make you sterile, there is really nothing you can do in terms of lifestyle changes (diet, exercise and so on) that will reduce this risk. There are, however, other measures that may help. These are different for men and women.

For men, if there is a chance that treatment will affect your fertility, then you should always be offered the chance of sperm banking before you begin chemotherapy. This involves giving several samples of your sperm, which are then frozen and stored. Sometimes the presence of the cancer actually reduces the number and quality of your sperm, but – even so – having your sperm stored is worthwhile because it may still be possible to use it to produce a pregnancy in the future, although success cannot be guaranteed. Incidentally, not having sex for a couple of days before you give the sperm samples will increase the quality of your specimen. Unfortunately, freezing the sperm does further reduce the quality of the sperm, but once they are frozen they can be kept indefinitely without any further deterioration. When you and your partner are finally ready to contemplate having children, your sperm can be thawed and used (this will involve some form of artificial insemination of your partner).

The rules vary from hospital to hospital, but you may find that there is a charge for the storage of your sperm.

For women the options are more limited. It is possible to freeze and store embryos that can later be thawed and re-implanted into the womb after treatment, but delaying your treatment long enough for this to be arranged will not usually be advisable. Even if you do go through this process, the chances of a successful pregnancy are probably still only about one in five. Having an operation to remove eggs (oocytes) from the ovary that are then frozen, and taking away pieces of ovarian tissue for storage that could be replaced after treatment to try to make the ovaries work again are both possible. However, these are really experimental approaches that are under development; at the moment, they have very little chance of success. Another option that you could consider is egg donation, where – after your treatment is over – your womb could be implanted with eggs given by another woman. This has resulted in successful pregnancies for some women after their ovaries have failed as result of chemotherapy.

Many types of chemotherapy will reduce fertility – lowering sperm counts in men or stopping periods in women – while you are actually on treatment but without resulting in permanent infertility. But it may take anywhere from six months to two years for your testicular or ovarian function to get back to normal. Usually, however, doctors would advise against having children during the first year after your treatment, so this possible delay should not be too much of a problem.

If your fertility is reduced but returns after chemotherapy, or if it was unaffected by treatment, then the drugs that you have had will not lead to any increase in the chances of birth defects in children that you may father or give birth to in the future. So it will be perfectly safe to have children as soon as your doctors think it is OK from the point of view of your cancer and its treatment.

Menopausal symptoms

Many women having hormonal treatments for breast cancer will develop menopausal symptoms. These can vary a great deal in the severity and the upset that they cause. They may involve no more than an occasional hot flush or there might be a combination of mood swings, irritability, finding it hard to concentrate, memory loss, difficulty in sleeping, vaginal dryness, loss of interest in sex, and severe hot flushes and drenching sweats that can drive a woman to the brink of suicide. A variety of things can be done to try to ease these symptoms, and because some degree of menopausal change is a very common problem we will look at these in more detail.

If the symptoms are due to taking tamoxifen, then changing the way the drug is taken might make a difference – either altering the time of day that you take it, or breaking the tablet in two and taking half in the morning and half at night. Tamoxifen is made by a number of different manufacturers, and although all of these products contain the same active drug some women find that changing from one brand of tamoxifen to another does make a difference and eases their menopausal problems. If none of these help, then for those women who are past their menopause a change from tamoxifen to an aromatase inhibitor, such as anastrozole (Arimidex), letrozole (Femara) or exemestane (Aromasin), might well help and will not make treatment any less effective.

Sometimes, simple lifestyle changes can help. Regular exercise, losing weight and avoiding certain foods (particularly spicy foods) and certain drinks (especially alcohol) may help to reduce the problem.

Complementary therapies may also make a difference. A number of preparations are available from local chemists and health food shops that include plant extracts containing a natural equivalent of the female hormone oestrogen. The active ingredients include red clover, soy, genistein and black cohosh. Some people have worried that because these compounds include a form of oestrogen they might increase the risk of breast cancer recurrence, but there is no evidence that this is the case. Evening primrose oil, ginseng and vitamin E supplements are other popular remedies, and many women feel that they reduce the number and severity of hot flushes and sweats, although scientific evidence for this is doubtful. Studies have shown, however, that both acupuncture and relaxation therapies can help some women.

Sometimes prescription drugs may improve things. The options here include low doses of the female hormone progesterone, certain types of antidepressants and a drug called clonidine (which alters the way the blood vessels work, sometimes easing the problem of hot flushes). None of these is a sure way of improving the problem, but if the symptoms are severe and troublesome it could be a good idea to have a word with your doctor to see whether they might be worth trying.

The role of hormone replacement therapy (HRT) is controversial. Certainly, it is often very effective at relieving the symptoms, but there are questions about its safety. At least one large clinical trial has shown that women who use HRT after a diagnosis of breast cancer have an increased risk of recurrence of their cancer, but this risk only seems to affect women over 50. So up to that age HRT may safely be given but thereafter – unless symptoms are very severe and all else has failed – HRT is not recommended

Bone thinning (osteoporosis)

This can be a problem if you take one of the aromatase inhibitor drugs anastrozole (Arimidex), letrozole (Femara) or exemestane (Aromasin) for more than a few months. Although there are no definitive national guidelines in the UK, it is generally suggested that women who are going to receive one of the aromatase inhibitors should have a special scan done to check the thickness of the bone in their spine and hips (this is called a bone densitometry, or DXA, scan) before treatment is started. Depending on the result of this scan, women may simply need advice on changes in lifestyle to reduce the risk of bone thinning (such as stopping smoking, reducing alcohol intake, taking regular exercise and eating a healthy diet) or they may be advised to take vitamin D and calcium supplements. For a few women who are at high risk, adding a bisphosphonate (see 'A note about bisphosphonates' in Chapter 3, page 25) to help strengthen their bones may be a wise precaution.

Hormonal therapies for prostate cancer

Most of the hormonal treatments used for prostate cancer can cause hot flushes and sweats, like those that women have when they go through the menopause. If these are troublesome, current guidelines from NICE recommend treatment with a synthetic female hormone, progestin, as the best remedy (this can be taken either as tablets or by injection). If this does not help then other prescription drugs such as clonidine or an antidepressant may be of some benefit but you will need to discuss this with your medical team. Alternatively, some of the lifestyle changes mentioned in the section on 'Menopausal symptoms' (see page 65) might make a difference.

A number of the hormonal drugs used to treat prostate cancer, but not usually bicalutamide (Casodex) and flutamide (Drogenil), can lead to a loss of libido and impotence, with difficulty in getting an erection. Once again, a change in treatment might help, but if this is not possible then ways of coping with the problems of loss of sex drive and erectile difficulties are discussed in Chapter 7.

The drugs bicalutamide (Casodex) and flutamide (Drogenil) may cause some breast enlargement and breast pain as well as 'menopausal' hot flushes. The risk of this happening can be reduced by giving a very low dose of radiotherapy to each breast before you start taking the drugs. Taking a single tablet of tamoxifen once a week may also prevent the breast pain and enlargement, and can sometimes help to control any breast discomfort that does develop as a result of bicalutamide or flutamide therapy.

If you have advanced prostate cancer, which has spread to your bones, and you are going to be given either goserelin (Zoladex), leuprorelin (Prostap) or triptorelin (Decapeptyl, Gonapeptyl), then there is a risk that for a short time they could actually make your symptoms worse before they get better (doctors call this a tumour flare). This can be prevented by giving you one of the anti-androgen drugs (usually either bicalutamide [Casodex] or flutamide [Drogenil]) as well for the first two or three weeks of treatment.

Targeted therapies

The targeted therapies include a number of different types of drug with a wide range of possible side effects. But the good news is that, compared with cytotoxic drugs, these side effects are generally much less troublesome and serious.

One of the more serious problems is the increased risk of heart failure caused by trastuzumab (Herceptin). This only occurs in a small number of people given this drug, and usually tests will be done to make sure your heart is healthy before it is given, which greatly reduces the risk. If heart failure does occur then it usually gets better rapidly with treatment, and stopping trastuzumab seems to reverse the problem, without leaving any long-term damage to the heart.

A number of the targeted therapies that have to be given by intravenous infusion (through a drip) can cause allergic reactions. If your medical team do feel there is a chance that this might happen, then they will usually give you some steroid tablets or other medication to take before you have the drip, which should prevent any hypersensitivity reactions.

Skin rashes

Skin rashes are quite common with a number of the targeted therapies. As a general rule, using mild soaps and moisturizers will help to ease any irritation or discomfort from the rash, but do get the advice of your medical team. Depending on the exact type of skin reaction you develop, it may be that prescription medicines – such as certain antibiotics or steroid creams – may improve things for you, and your doctors and specialist nurses will be able to point you in the right direction. Many of these rashes are only temporary and settle after a week or two on treatment, disappearing completely even though you are continuing with the drug.

7

Other ways to cope with chemotherapy

In this chapter we will look at some more general ways of helping you to cope with chemotherapy.

The spiritual dimension

For many people their religious faith can give valuable support during the stresses and strains of cancer treatment. This spiritual dimension often provides comfort and reassurance, and gives emotional strength to work through the more difficult days. Prayer and belief will offer hope and meaning when times are bad.

This is a very personal subject, and the beliefs that each of us hold will vary in their nature and in their importance to us. But one general point to make is that, like everything else we will discuss in this chapter, your faith should be used as a means of support during your chemotherapy and not as an alternative to it. Spiritual strength can make living with the effects of chemotherapy easier – it may even increase the chances of successful treatment – but it cannot take the place of conventional medicine: the two should always work together.

Talking

Talking can be very helpful. That does not mean it is always easy.

Talking about your treatment and your cancer can have many benefits. Sharing your experiences, concerns, worries and problems can be very positive. That is not to say that other people will always have answers, although sometimes they might, but simply expressing your feelings can help. It can help because it lets you begin to work out what your concerns are, what things you need to know or do, what questions you need to ask and what support you might need. Just explaining things that may be troubling you can often make them less troubling and sometimes reassure you that your fears are unfounded. Talking things through may help you to appreciate that something you thought would be a major issue in your case is unlikely to happen or can be handled relatively easily.

Talking also helps you to gain a sense of control over your situation. It helps you to sort out what things are important to you personally, both positively (things you want to do and achieve) and negatively (things you are worried might happen). You can then decide which of these are the most important, and form a plan to do the things you want to do and find out about and cope with the things that are causing you concern.

Bottling things up, keeping things to yourself, can often make matters worse. When thoughts go round and round in our heads our fears can often get out of proportion – the worry just goes on growing. But by sharing your anxieties, bringing things out into the open, that vicious circle can often be broken. Although the basic problem may not go away, it can become much easier to live with.

Sometimes, just explaining things and being reassured that the feelings you have are quite natural in your situation can be therapeutic, letting you know that your sensations and emotions are normal and understandable under the circumstances.

There is always the question of who to talk to. A caring and sympathetic partner is the obvious choice – someone who knows you and cares deeply about your well-being and who, even if they cannot change things, can listen with understanding and appreciate how you are feeling. But not everyone has such a partner, or you may feel that talking in this way is placing too great a burden on your partner, although very often these sorts of conversations can actually strengthen the bonds of your relationship and bring you even closer together.

But if talking to your nearest and dearest is something you find difficult, then it may be easier to talk to someone on your medical team. The people you are likely to see most of the time during your treatment are your chemotherapy nurses, and it is likely that you will get to know one or two of them very well during your time on treatment. If you ask them they will often be able to find the time to chat about your worries with you. Once again, they may often be able to reassure you that things you are frightened about are unlikely to happen, or give you good advice on how to reduce the risk of them happening or cope with them if they do.

Some hospital departments actually have counsellors available who you can talk to about your illness and treatment, and all the emotional and practical concerns that they are causing. Another alternative that is sometimes possible is to meet and talk to other people who have had your type of cancer and similar treatment. They can tell you how they got on and how they managed the sort of issues you are facing. Often, this sort of opportunity is offered by cancer support groups (see page 81), where people who have or have had cancer (and their relatives and carers) can meet on a regular basis and discuss their experiences. Discovering that other people have had similar thoughts and fears to yours can often be very comforting, allowing you to realize that the issues you are facing are not something you have to confront alone. You can share your experiences with others and sometimes learn from theirs.

Although these sorts of exchanges can sometimes be very valuable, it is important to remember that each of us is a unique individual. Even when someone has had the same type of cancer as you and had treatment nearly the same as yours, their experiences might differ. They may have had different side effects, feelings about everything that was going on, worries and solutions. So do not expect that everything that happened to them will happen to you in the same way.

If you do want to talk about things, do let people know. Very often, family and friends will be worried that asking you about your condition, how you are feeling and how things are going will upset you. They might even think that *not* talking about what is going on will be doing you a kindness, sparing you distress. So if you want to talk about your treatment or your cancer, do not hesitate to bring the subject up. Bringing things out into the open will often create a much more relaxed atmosphere all round among those who are close to you. Equally, if there are times when you don't want to talk, when you just want a bit of peace or when going over things again will be too much, then say so. Let people know when you need some time to yourself, to get your thoughts in order, or just to get away from it all for a while. You are the one having chemotherapy, so take control and talk as much or as little as you want to.

Diet – what to eat

There is a huge amount of information – and misinformation – about diet and cancer. Every week stories appear in the newspapers, in magazines and on the television about this or that food which is either good or bad, and there are countless suggestions for diets that will help prevent or fight the disease.

In trying to make sense of all this confusing – and often conflicting – advice, the first step is to realize that there are two completely separate questions when it comes to the subject of food and cancer. First, can what we eat increase or reduce our risk of getting cancer? Second, once someone has cancer can their diet increase their chances of being cured?

There is now good scientific evidence that what people eat does alter their chances of getting some types of cancer. For example, high consumption of red meat increases the risk of getting two of the commonest types of cancer: bowel cancer and prostate cancer. On the other hand there are many myths about diet and cancer risk. For instance, there is a popular belief that high intake of dairy products increases the risk of getting breast cancer, but there is no real evidence for this (although being overweight does increase a woman's chances of getting the disease). On the positive side there are also foods that can help to reduce the likelihood of developing cancer. A diet rich in fibre (with plenty of fruit and vegetables) makes bowel cancer less likely, and plenty of fish and tomato is linked to a lower risk of prostate cancer.

But these things all relate to preventing or avoiding cancer in the first place. It is thought that the foods that are linked to cancer development will, over a period of time, help to trigger changes in the cells that make them cancerous. Once that change has taken place and the cancer has begun to grow, however, there is virtually no evidence that a change in diet can slow down or reverse the cancer's progression. So once someone actually has a cancer, changing their diet is not going to influence how rapidly or slowly the tumour grows, and is not going to make any difference to whether they will be cured.

Despite this there are countless recommendations given in the media, on websites, at independent, non-NHS clinics, and by well-meaning people everywhere for diets that will help to make the cancer better. Many people believe passionately in these and are convinced of their benefits, but none has been shown scientifically to alter how a cancer will behave.

So when you are having chemotherapy, what you eat will make no difference to the chances of success of your treatment. It is very important to remember this, so that you can focus on what is really important about your diet during this time.

The two main things that are important about what you eat during chemotherapy are that you have what you enjoy and are comfortable with, and that you try and keep a healthy balance in your food.

When it comes to enjoying and being comfortable with what you eat, there are a number of things to remember. These include the following.

- It is quite likely that your tastes will change while you are going through chemotherapy. Some things you were fond of before may taste different, and even unpleasant, whereas things you didn't particularly like now seem very toothsome. So be prepared to vary your diet.
- Your appetite will vary a lot while you are on treatment, and it is likely that there will be times when you won't really fancy food. Generally speaking, having light meals or snacks and eating little and often is easier and pleasanter than having one or two big meals a day.
- Well meaning relatives and friends are likely to get anxious if they see that you are eating less, especially if you start to lose a bit of weight. But having people continually coaxing and encouraging you to have something can be very off-putting and

make you feel even less like eating. As long as you are drinking plenty, having the odd day or two when you don't eat very much is quite all right.

- Your system will probably cope best with foods that are easy to digest. So changing from red meats to things like chicken, eggs or fish, and avoiding heavy puddings, fatty pastries and rich sauces can all help. But if you do suddenly fancy something rich and stodgy, then go for it – eat what you enjoy.

For a healthy diet, the best overall advice is to have plenty of fresh fruit and vegetables, keep portions of red meat – especially processed meat (such as sausages, bacon and pies) – to two or three times a week, and to watch your salt intake. This not only is consistent with what evidence there is for the risks and benefits of diet and cancer, but it will also fit with the far stronger evidence for the ability of a healthy diet to reduce the risk of heart disease and diabetes.

Incidentally, the evidence is that if you have successfully come through your cancer treatment, then keeping to this sort of healthy diet does reduce the chances of your cancer coming back in the future.

Some of the 'cancer diets' that you may come across recommend ridiculous amounts of certain things – at least 500 grams of grated raw carrot every day or masses of lightly steamed broccoli, or limitless quantities of raw blueberries. Don't be dictated to by these recommendations; having a selection of fresh fruit and vegetables on a regular basis is what matters. Aiming for the Department of Health's target of five portions of fruit or vegetables every day is a good target but, once again, if you don't feel up to it then don't force yourself.

As far as fluid is concerned, try to aim for at least two litres (four pints) every day. Plenty of water is good for keeping the system flushed through, but any other drinks you fancy are OK. Incidentally, many people worry about having alcohol while they are on chemotherapy. Certainly, getting drunk is not a good idea, but – except in rare circumstances – having a glass of wine or a pint of beer will not do any harm at all. In fact, alcohol can sometimes help if your appetite is low; a glass of sherry, and particularly dry sherry, about 15 minutes before you are due to eat can often stimulate digestion and make food more appealing.

Most cancer chemotherapy departments have specially trained dieticians who work with them. So if during your treatment you are worried about what you should eat and drink, or if you find that you are losing more weight than you are comfortable with, then do ask to have a word with them so that you can get expert professional advice.

Exercise

We are constantly being told that regular exercise is good for us, and this is true. But when you are having chemotherapy you will often feel worn out and probably not very well. The thought of rushing off to the gym or going for a quick jog round the block is unlikely to be high on your list of priorities.

Exercise can make you feel better. It helps to fight off depression, it can improve your appetite and reduce the risk of constipation, and it lowers your chances of getting blood clots in your veins (thrombosis). It is also a way to take your mind off things for a while – a distraction from everything else that is going on.

The secret of exercise during chemotherapy is achieving a personal balance. Trying to force yourself to do vigorous activities that you can't face is just as bad as simply retreating to bed and giving up. The key word to go with 'exercise' in this situation is 'gentle'. Do enough to keep your body mobile and in reasonable shape. Keep in trim by basing your activities on what you did before you started the treatment. If you used to run ten miles a day in training for a half-marathon, then cut back to a regular trot round the park; if all you managed was four trips up and down stairs each day, then still try to make that short journey a couple of times a day. Don't push yourself unduly and don't try to take on strenuous new activities because you feel you have to, but equally don't stop everything.

It is often said that walking is the best exercise, and this is probably true during your treatment. If you can manage a short walk, stroll or amble about each day, then this will keep your system ticking over. It can also provide you with a period of time when you can get out of the house and have a bit of a change of scene.

Complementary therapies

Complementary therapies can be used alongside conventional treatments, such as surgery, radiotherapy or chemotherapy, to help people to cope with their illness. They are not intended to cure the cancer but are used to ease any side effects of treatment and improve general well-being.

This is different from alternative therapies, which are unconventional treatments given to try to control or cure the cancer. Alternative therapies are often recommended with claims for activity and benefit that sound convincing but have no medical proof. Sometimes they have actually been shown to be ineffective, or even harmful, but are still being promoted to unsuspecting members of the public. They frequently involve considerable expense and insist on demanding changes in lifestyle, with outlandish diets or special supplements of 'essential elements', 'vital vitamins' or 'immunity-boosting drugs' – none of which have ever been scientifically proven to work.

This contrasts with many complementary therapies, which are generally used alongside mainstream medical care, and which are safe, well understood, can actually be pleasant to have and usually have a positive effect on well-being.

Although health professionals remain highly unconvinced of the claims made by alternative therapies, their attitude to complementary therapies has changed greatly over the past ten years. More and more doctors and nurses have come to view them as useful additions to conventional therapies that very often can improve the quality of life of their patients. Combining conventional and complementary therapies can frequently be a productive partnership.

Many people try complementary therapies while they are having chemotherapy. The main types of complementary therapies are the touch therapies (aromatherapy, massage therapy, reflexology and acupuncture), fitness and movement therapies (yoga, t'ai chi and qigong), psychological therapies (relaxation, meditation, visualization and music therapy) and diet.

Aromatherapy involves the use of essential oils. These are plant extracts that have distinctive smells. Each of the different essential oils is believed to have particular physical or psychological effects, for example lavender and eucalyptus help to ease stress, whereas camomile reduces inflammation. The oils may be used in massage, given as inhalations or aromatic baths, or applied as creams or lotions. Reflexology is based on the belief that areas on the feet match different parts of the body, and by applying pressure to these areas energy paths are triggered that can produce beneficial effects. It is a type of foot massage. Acupuncture is based on ancient Chinese medicine, which believes that the body's energy, or *chi*, moves in pathways, or meridians, beneath the skin. By inserting needles into these meridians a healing response can be stimulated.

Aromatherapy and reflexology are very relaxing, and many people with cancer say that they feel better after having these treatments. Acupuncture is rather more uncomfortable, but there is some evidence that it can help to ease pain and sickness if these are a problem. At the present time there is very little scientific evidence for the value of these different therapies, although an increasing number of clinical trials using these treatments are under way, and there is a growing belief that they can be helpful.

The fitness and movement therapies do involve more active participation, rather than just lying back and enjoying the therapy. But many people do find that they can help to ease anxiety and depression, as well as giving a bit of gentle exercise to keep up overall fitness.

The psychological therapies can be as simple as just relaxing in a quiet room listening to restful music, or they might involve working with a counsellor who teaches you relaxation techniques or uses visualization (picturing your body and how it is working to fight the cancer or reduce the side effects of treatment). Art therapy and music therapy, using drawing or painting to channel your emotions or listening to (and sometimes taking part in) live music performances, are other approaches to psychological therapy. Many people find that these techniques can help to ease stress and anxiety and make them feel better during their treatment.

Dietary changes may involve simply taking one or more supplements to your normal diet, or a complete change in the way you eat. This is one area in which the boundaries between complementary and alternative therapies become blurred. There are many people who claim that particular diets or supplements will help to ease the side effects of treatment and sometimes suggest that they will actually help to control the cancer or prevent it coming back. Very often these claims are based on the belief that the change in diet will boost the immune system. Unfortunately, there is virtually no evidence to support any of these claims. Also, occasionally these diets can be quite extreme and unpleasant (or expensive), and actually reduce your quality of life rather than enhancing it. Having a normal balanced range of foods – with plenty of fresh fruit and vegetables – is very hard to beat.

Complementary therapies can have a lot of appeal. They often lead to emotional and spiritual well-being, with relief from stress and anxiety, and they may actually reduce some of the side effects of treatment or make them easier to live with. They also offer some empowerment. It is one part of your treatment and overall care that you can take control of and decide exactly how and when you want to use it. This is particularly valuable at a time when – with a cancer diagnosis and all the tests and treatments that follow – it can seem that the running of everyday life has gone completely out of your hands.

Each of us is different, and with complementary therapies people vary greatly in their responses. How much they will help in coping with the stresses and strains of chemotherapy, and how much they will relieve any side effects such as tiredness or sickness varies hugely from one person to another. Some people will feel a real benefit whereas others won't notice any difference. If you want to try any of these therapies, do check first with your medical team that it is all right for you to do so, and then give it a try. If you find that you enjoy it and feel better for it, then that is great, but if it doesn't help then don't hesitate to stop. Sometimes, particularly with diets, people start on a new regime and find that they really don't like it but feel they must continue or they will get worse. This is not what complementary therapies are about – they are there to improve your quality of life, not reduce it. And if you do try a new diet, or any other type of complementary therapy, and find that you feel more miserable as a result, then do stop it at once.

Times are changing. Conventional doctors are becoming more sympathetic toward complementary therapies, and some cancer centres will offer these as part of their service to NHS patients. But unfortunately the availability of these services in hospitals or general practitioners' surgeries is still very patchy and variable. It is likely that if you do want to pursue any of these options, then you will have to make your own arrangements and pay for them.

Information

For many people, simply understanding what is going on – what is happening to them – is a very important part of being able to cope with difficult situations such as cancer and chemotherapy. That means knowledge, which in turn means information.

Your doctors and nurses should keep you fully informed of everything about your illness and its treatment. Sometimes they don't, however, and even when they do there may be things you want to know more about.

Information comes in many different forms. The simple chat with your medical team can be very helpful but leaves you with nothing to refer to afterward. So more and more often nowadays, these conversations are being backed up by leaflets, booklets or DVDs that you can take away and look at later. Then there are books (like this one!) and, of course, the internet.

There is a vast amount of information out there dealing with every aspect of cancer and its treatment that you could possibly think of. The two problems are getting hold of that information and knowing whether it is reliable. The Department of Health is very keen for people with cancer to have as much information as they want, and so your medical team should welcome any questions you have about where to get this and be able to point you in the right direction. They may offer leaflets or booklets that they have produced themselves, or provide literature from approved organizations such as Macmillan Cancer Support or Cancer Research UK. They can also give you the contact details to reach these organizations' websites, where you will find a wealth of information. More details about these organizations and their contact details are given in the Useful addresses section at the end of this book. You are perfectly free to get in touch with any of these groups yourself, and you do not need the approval of your doctors first.

Incidentally, in the past Cancerbackup was the foremost charity for providing information for people with cancer and their carers. In 2008 Cancerbackup merged with Macmillan Cancer Support, and all its various information resources – booklets, leaflets, helpline and website – are now available through Macmillan.

Although there is limitless good and reliable coverage of all aspects of cancer on the internet, there is also a huge amount of misinformation, some of which is not only misleading but down-right dangerous. Just because something is on the internet does not mean it can be believed, even though it may look and sound very convincing.

Cancer support groups

Another source of both support and information can be a local cancer support group. These developed informally during the 1980s and have grown in number since. They have no fixed pattern, and so they vary very much from place to place. Sometimes they are run by specialist nurses from the hospital (in which case they often focus on one particular type of cancer), or they may be based in the community, associated with a local health centre, a church or a community centre. What the various groups do have in common is that they provide an opportunity to meet other people in a similar situation to yours or who have been through the same sort of experience in the past, so that you can compare and contrast views in a social setting. There is often some form of professional input, with informal talks from experts in various fields on one or other aspect of the subject, and there is likely to be a supply of suitable background information or someone who can give advice on where to get such information. There may also be other activities; for instance, some complementary therapies may be available, as may access to spiritual support from local faith leaders.

The availability of cancer support groups and the format of the groups varies from place to place, but if the idea interests you then do ask your doctors and nurses about it. They should be able to let you know what is on offer in your area.

8

Chemotherapy and everyday life

Although it may change, your everyday life does not stop while you are having chemotherapy. Work and holidays, money and sex, and friends and neighbours are all parts of day to day living that might be affected by your treatment. This chapter explains some of the problems you might face and offers some advice to help you cope with them.

Work and chemotherapy

The effect of chemotherapy on someone's lifestyle will depend on the type of treatment they need and their individual reactions to that treatment. For a few people chemotherapy will have little or no impact on their day to day life, but for others – who need intensive treatment over a long time – their lives will change completely.

A typical course of chemotherapy will involve treatment over four to six months. Even if you have few obviously troublesome side effects during this time, it is likely that the treatment will make you feel more tired than usual. You are also likely to have lots of visits to the hospital, not only for the chemotherapy itself but also for blood tests and check-ups. Once the chemotherapy has actually finished, it is quite likely that the feeling of fatigue will last for some months afterward.

These various disruptions caused by the treatment do mean that carrying on working while you are having chemotherapy is very difficult for most people. So, if you are working and facing the prospect of having chemotherapy, then you need to think ahead about how this will affect your job.

Some basic facts about your cancer and its treatment will help with your planning, so you should ask your doctors and nurses some of the following questions.

- How long will the chemotherapy go on for?
- What will be involved, in terms of the number and frequency of hospital visits?
- What are the likely side effects, how troublesome might they be and how long are they likely to last?
- What is the likely outcome of the treatment? Will the cancer probably be cured completely, or is the chemotherapy intended to control it for a period of time before it comes back again?

Of course, you can also get their advice on how easy or difficult they feel it might be for you to carry on working during treatment.

Once you have this information, you can start to think about what you would like to do with respect to your job. For some people, work is the most important thing in their life and they would do anything possible to avoid having time off. For others, work is a drudge and a chore, and the chance to give it up – even for a while – would be a real bonus. Also, for some people the diagnosis of cancer and its treatment might give them the opportunity for early retirement, or retirement on the grounds of ill health, and this may be something else you might want to think about.

When you have an idea of how you would like to handle your working life during and immediately after chemotherapy, the next thing is to talk to your employer about the options available. Most employers will be sympathetic in this situation, and try and make arrangements for things like time off, flexible working hours, lighter duties or working from home. If your workplace has an occupational health department or a human resources team, then chatting to them can often give you a good idea of the choices open to you. They will be able to tell you about your company's sickness policies and your entitlements to sick leave, and pay during that time. They will also treat their discussions with you in strict confidence.

Most employers are very supportive of members of staff who develop cancer and need chemotherapy. But if you do have problems, then you also do have rights. Most people with cancer will be covered by the Disability Discrimination Act. This Act says that it is unlawful for an employer to discriminate against a person because of their disability. To be classed as 'disabled' under the Act, someone with cancer must have symptoms or side effects of treatment that interfere with their day to day activities. Therefore, if the effects of your chemotherapy mean that your treatment will limit your ability to work, or prevent you from working at all, then you should be covered. The Act also covers people who have recovered from a disability, so if you have been cured as a result of your treatment then your employer cannot discriminate against you because you have had cancer in the past.

Under the terms of the Act an employer should make 'reasonable adjustments' to workplaces and working practices to make sure that you are not at any substantial disadvantage relative to your colleagues. The phrase 'reasonable adjustments' would usually cover things like time off for hospital visits, changes in your working hours, avoiding physically demanding jobs or allowing a gradual return to work after a period of sick leave.

If you feel your supervisors or managers are being unreasonable or unhelpful, then you could talk to your occupational health or human resources team at work. If you need advice from outside your workplace, then you could talk to your union representative or contact your local Citizens Advice Bureau. Very occasionally, it may even help to get guidance from a lawyer.

Financial help

In 2004 a survey by Macmillan Cancer Support suggested that more than three out four people in the UK diagnosed with cancer suffered some financial hardship. In 2008 the same charity estimated that of the 1.2 million people in Britain living with the consequences of cancer, some 400,000 were likely to need guidance in managing their finances and making ends meet. There is a lot of help on offer for people with cancer, but there is evidence that this help is often not taken up. One estimate suggests that every year more than £126 million in state benefits are not claimed by cancer patients who are entitled to them. A number of the national cancer charities have leaflets or booklets on financial problems, and Macmillan Cancer Support is particularly active in this area. They have a free booklet called 'Helping with the cost of cancer', which you can get by ringing their free hotline on 0808 808 00 00 or visiting <www .macmillan.org.uk>.

Managing your personal finances

It may be that you have been lucky and that your cancer and its chemotherapy treatment have had very little impact on your day-to-day life. But if your circumstances have changed and your income has been affected, you may need to look at some aspects of the way in which you manage your money. This might include reviewing things such as insurance, retirement and pensions, mortgages, loans and the possibility of outside help with grants.

If you have insurance policies that relate to your general health and fitness, it is worth looking at what they cover, and checking with your insurance company whether you are entitled to make a claim. The type of policies that might be relevant include income protection, critical illness cover and some private medical insurance schemes. If you have private medical insurance as part of your employment package, then it is possible that there might be some benefits you could claim from this. Your manager or your company's human resources team might be able to advise you about this.

For most of us our mortgage is the major financial burden we have to carry and the main drain on our monthly income. If mortgage repayments are a problem, check whether you have any insurance policies linked to your mortgage that might give you some protection and cover some of the costs. If not, then it may be possible to agree a lower monthly rate of repayment by re-mortgaging at a lower rate or extending the period of your borrowing, especially if you have already paid off some of the capital on your property (so that you have equity in your property). Alternatively, you may be able to change to a loan based on interest payments only for a period of time. The key thing here is to let your lender know about your change in circumstances and talk to them about the options available to you.

On a similar theme, look at all your regular outgoings – payments that are made weekly, monthly or once a year – and check whether any of these can be stopped or reduced. For example, subscriptions to organizations you are no longer interested in, insurance policies that are no longer necessary or charitable donations you can no longer afford. If you are facing a short-term problem in your finances, then it is sometimes possible to agree deferred payments for things such as rent, council tax and energy bills, giving you a few months to get your income sorted out. Talk to your landlord, local council and energy supplier to see whether they offer such schemes. Similarly, if you have outstanding loans on credit cards or store cards, check whether these can be swapped to companies charging lower interest rates or whether you can negotiate a lower rate of monthly repayments.

State benefits

The benefits system is complicated and confusing, and many people simply don't make a claim because they do not realize what they are entitled to. Other people simply feel embarrassed about taking 'charity' or asking for help. But these benefits are yours by right, and if you are eligible then you should not hesitate to take advantage of them.

The benefits system is quite regularly changed or adjusted, so the following account gives an overview of what was available in early 2009, but you should check to make sure that things haven't changed. Some benefits are means tested and only given to people on lower incomes or with little in the way of savings, but others are more widely available. These include Statutory Sick Pay, Employment and Support Allowance, Disability Living Allowance and Attendance Allowance.

Statutory Sick Pay

If you have been working and making National Insurance contributions then you should receive Statutory Sick Pay from your employer for the first 28 weeks you are off sick (this may be a continuous period of sick leave or a number of episodes relating to the same illness). You need to let your employer know about your illness and give them a doctor's certificate after your first week off work. Your employer will then pay you at the Statutory Sick Pay level in the same way as they paid your salary. This is a minimum payment determined by the Government but your employment contract may guarantee a more generous allowance, so do check on this. If you are still not back at work after 28 weeks then you can claim Employment and Support Allowance.

The Employment and Support Allowance

This was introduced in October 2008 and replaced the previous Incapacity Benefit and Income Support (people who were on those benefits before October 2008 were not affected and continue to receive the old allowances).

People who want to claim this allowance will have to undergo an assessment carried out by a health professional, on behalf of the Department of Work and Pensions, to see whether their ability to work is reduced. They must also satisfy one of the following conditions.

- They have paid enough National Insurance to qualify for the benefit.
- They are under 20 years old (or 25 if they have been in education or training).
- They are on a low income.

These various conditions do not apply to those who are considered to be terminally ill.

Full information about this new benefit is available from the Department of Work and Pensions (<www.dwp.gov.uk/esa>).

Disability Living Allowance

Disability Living Allowance is for people under the age of 65 who need help with their care, and this includes people who are left with a disability as a result of their cancer or the side effects of treatment. The allowance is based on the level of your disability and is not related to your National Insurance contributions or any other income or savings you may have; it is also tax free. There is a time factor in that you usually need to have had your disability for at least three months, and it is likely to continue for at least another six months. You can claim Disability Living Allowance even if you are still able to work, and even if you do not have anyone to give you the care that you need. (In other words, you don't have to have a carer to get the allowance.) The allowance is paid at several different levels depending on your degree of disability and your needs, which are grouped under two headings: the care component and the mobility component. If you get Disability Living Allowance under the mobility component then you will also get the Blue Badge, giving free parking in most places and free road tax.

If you are entitled to Disability Living Allowance it is likely that your medical team will have all the necessary information to help you claim it, but if not you can get claim forms from your local Social Security office.

Attendance Allowance

This is broadly similar to Disability Living Allowance but is for people over the age of 65.

Means-tested benefits

There are a wide range of benefits available to people who are on low incomes or with little or no savings. The type of benefit and the amount you receive varies with your individual circumstances. These benefits include Pension Credit and Jobseeker's Allowance. There are also tax credits from the Inland Revenue including Child Tax Credit and Working Tax Credit. Then there are benefits from your local council, including Council Tax Benefit, Housing Benefit, free school meals and grants for children over 16 who are continuing in full-time education. You may also be eligible for help with travel costs to hospital.

Having so many different benefits and allowances makes it quite a daunting task to find out just what is available and what you are entitled to. The Citizens Advice Bureau is very good at helping you through the maze of benefit options, or you could contact your local Social Security office or ring the Benefit Enquiry Line (0800 882200).

Incidentally, if you have been claiming benefits and then decide to go back to work, this can affect your entitlements. Disability Living Allowance and Attendance Allowance are both paid whether you are working or not, and if you go back to work but your earnings are small then you may still be able to claim any means-tested benefits. But Incapacity Benefit stops if you return to work, although if you find that you are not coping and have to give up work again you can restart the benefit, at the same rate, provided you apply within 56 days from the time you stopped it.

Prescription charges

After years of campaigning by patient advocacy groups, the Department of Health announced that from 1 April 2009 people with cancer do not have to pay prescription charges. This includes people who are having treatment for the effects of cancer (such as pain or sickness) or the side effects of cancer treatment, as well as treatment for the cancer itself. To get this benefit you have to have an Exemption Certificate, which has to be signed by a doctor, and the necessary forms should be available from either your family doctor or your hospital medical team. The Exemption Certificate lasts for five years and covers all prescription charges, not just those related to your cancer. So, for example, if you have tablets for high blood pressure you do not have to pay for these.

Devolution means that the rules and regulations vary in different parts of the UK. In Wales all prescription charges were withdrawn in 2007; in Northern Ireland prescriptions have cost £3 each since January 2009 and should be free from April 2010; and in Scotland charges are being phased out by 2011.

Holidays and travel

The fact that most chemotherapy treatments are given every few weeks means that it is sometimes possible to go away for a short holiday between courses. If you are thinking of having a short break somewhere in Britain, this is usually fairly straightforward, but a holiday abroad may be more difficult.

For a trip in the UK the first thing to do is to check with your doctors and nurses that they think it will be safe for you to do this, and that it won't interfere with any treatment or tests that you need. Once you have their agreement, then the two things you need to make sure of are that you have a good supply of all the medicines you need, or might need, and that you have some written information about your cancer and its treatment. This is a wise precaution, because if you were to be taken ill and had difficulty in getting straight back to your own hospital, then the doctors where you were staying would need to have details about your condition and the drugs you were having, so that they could take care of you. These days most people having chemotherapy will have their own handheld record books, giving all the necessary information and contact details, so taking this would be the ideal. If you don't have your own record book, then ask your doctor or nurses for a letter that gives all the relevant information you need to take with you.

Holidays abroad present more problems. Even if your medical team are happy for you to travel overseas, you may have difficulty getting travel insurance. Most insurers will be reluctant to insure people who are having chemotherapy or who are within a month or so of having completed their treatment. Some insurers also refuse cover if you have recently had a blood transfusion. It is worth shopping around, however, because companies do vary and you may find that you will be able to get cover, although you may have to pay a premium, and they might also want a report from your doctor confirming that it is all right for you to go abroad.

Planning for overseas trips

- As with UK trips, taking written details of your cancer and its treatment is essential.
- Do take a good supply of all the drugs you need (and take some extra in case of delays on your journey). If you have drugs that have to be given by injection, requiring needles and syringes, or if you are taking narcotic drugs such as morphine, then you may need special permission from the immigration services of the country you are going to and special documents from your doctors. Your travel company should be able to advise you, or you could contact the embassy of the country you are hoping to visit.
- Many people with cancer have a higher than normal risk of deep vein thrombosis, and this risk is further increased if you are on certain drugs such as tamoxifen. So if you are going on a long-haul flight, check with your doctors to see whether they feel that you are at risk and what precautions you ought to take.
- If you are hoping to go to somewhere where you need vaccinations, this could be a problem. Because of the reduced immunity caused by chemotherapy, some vaccines might actually be dangerous and others could be ineffective. Once again, have a chat with your doctor if you are going to need vaccinations.

Getting insurance is often easier if you are travelling to countries within the European Union, or certain other countries that have reciprocal health agreements with the UK, which mean that any treatment you have there would either be free or relatively cheap. By contrast, countries where health costs are much higher – like the USA – would be more difficult to get insurance for.

If you are going abroad and you have insurance, then there are a few other things to bear in mind (see the information box 'Planning for overseas trips'.)

Sex

Sex is a sensitive and very personal subject. This means that it is often something that people starting chemotherapy feel shy about discussing with their doctors and nurses. Because it is not talked about very much, people do often worry so it is important to start by stating a few facts.

First, no one can catch cancer from someone else by having sex with them. So there is no risk that you could pass on your cancer to your partner by carrying on with your normal love life. Second, having sex does not make the cancer worse or – if it has already been removed – increase the risk of it coming back. Third, having sex won't interfere with your chemotherapy. It won't stop the drugs from working or make them any less effective or increase the risk of side effects. So sex is safe during chemotherapy.

Having said this, most doctors recommend that if you do make love while you are going through the treatment, it is a good idea to use a barrier form of protection, with a condom. There are several reasons for this.

- If you are a woman who has not yet gone through the menopause, you could still become pregnant while you are having chemotherapy, even if your periods have stopped as a result of the treatment. So you do still need some form of contraception.
- Although there is no very good evidence for it, many experts believe that small traces of the chemotherapy drugs, or chemicals formed by their breakdown in the body, can find their way into

the male semen or the female fluids that moisten the vagina, and these could cause soreness or discomfort to your partner.

Another word of caution is that if you are a woman and you have had surgery or radiotherapy to your pelvis as part of your treatment before chemotherapy, then you should check how soon it will be safe for you to restart penetrative sex. Your specialist nurses will usually discuss this with you as part of their care during your treatment.

Although there is no medical reason why you should not continue your normal love life during your treatment, many people simply don't feel like it. This may be due to a number of things.

- *Tiredness.* Feeling tired and completely drained of energy is the commonest of all of the side effects of chemotherapy, and most people just don't feel like having sex when they feel worn out.
- *Side effects.* The chemotherapy may cause other side effects that are upsetting and just make you feel miserable. No one is likely to enjoy sex if they are feeling nauseous.
- *Anxiety.* Being worried about your cancer and its treatment is very understandable, and if you are feeling anxious then you are likely to be less keen on sex.
- *Depression.* Sometimes natural anxiety tips over into clinical depression, feeling generally low and lacking interest in things generally, including love making.
- *Effects of the cancer.* If your cancer is still present then the illness itself may be making you feel unwell and switching off your interest.

Any or all of these things may affect your feelings about sex while you are having chemotherapy and for some time afterward.

The first and most important step in handling this change in your feelings is talking, and the most important person to talk to is your partner. Many people find that talking about sex, and in particular their own needs and emotions, is not easy. But letting your partner know what you are experiencing is essential, so that you can reach a shared understanding of the way you are feeling. Talking may be hard but it is far better than hiding your worries and concerns, or trying to pretend that things are normal when they are not.

Every relationship between two people is different and has a different mix of things that hold that relationship together. But love, mutual respect, and a desire to protect and care for your partner are common cores to most couples that can be drawn on. These should form the background that allows you to discuss difficult subjects with your partner in a positive way, whereas secrecy and uncertainty can be damaging.

Usually, partners will be understanding, supportive and sympathetic. So that once you bring up the subject of sex, finding ways to adapt to your altered desires and emotions should become easier. You will at least have created a starting point from which you can work together to address any problems in your relationship caused by your change in sexuality.

For some couples communication is more difficult, and even just starting to talk together about anything as sensitive as sex may be hard. If this is the case then counselling may help. A trained counsellor might well be able to help you overcome the reservations, inhibitions or anxieties that are holding back an open discussion of the subject. Furthermore, a counsellor might not only help you to identify the problems but also pave the way toward finding solutions. Quite a few hospitals do have counsellors available for their cancer patients, and there are also sources of help outside the NHS.

Once this background awareness of the situation has been established, you can go on to look at ways to cope with it.

The most likely difficulty is a mismatch in desire, with the person who is having treatment feeling less sexy, whereas their partner's libido remains much the same. This is very natural for both parties, and neither of you should be guilty about the way you are feeling. Once again, talking will help you to reach an understanding that your physical desires are different and that this difference is entirely reasonable. From that basis of acceptance of difference, you can begin to sort out how to handle the situation. The solutions will be different for different people. They might include an agreed abstinence, a period of celibacy until you both feel the time is right, or you might adjust your relationship to one of hugs, caresses and cuddles, showing your love physically without actual sex. Alternatively, you might change your approach to sex, with a greater emphasis on things like touching, stroking and masturbation, rather than penetrative sex, or changes in position that make actual intercourse more relaxed and less tiring.

These adjustments can only be made by you and your partner, and can only be achieved by talking and understanding. There are no rights or wrongs, no set rules for how the sexual dynamics of a couple should change at these times. So finding out what works for you is the right answer, rather than thinking that there is some magic formula that you ought to try and follow.

There are a few practical issues that are also worth mentioning.

Many women will find that they get vaginal soreness and dryness during their chemotherapy, which can make intercourse uncomfortable or even painful. Sometimes this can be due to fungal infection in the vagina, because of reduced immunity caused by chemotherapy. In this case the soreness is often accompanied by itching and irritation, and sometimes a white or yellowish vaginal discharge. If this does happen then a short course of antifungal drugs will usually clear this up very quickly, in a matter of a few days. So if you do suspect this problem, do mention it to your nurses or doctors. Vaginal dryness often develops during treatment because of hormonal changes caused by the chemotherapy. These may often be temporary and disappear a few months after treatment is over, but they can be unpleasant at the time. If vaginal dryness is a problem then there are a number of solutions. Various lubricants that you can buy at chemists or supermarkets, including KY Jelly, Senselle, Sylk and Astroglide, or simple glycerine can be used as an alternative (although glycerine, unlike the other lubricants, is not water soluble and so is a bit more sticky). Another alternative is Replens, which again can be bought over the counter. This gel is a longer acting vaginal moisturizer, and if it is used three times a week it can help to overcome vaginal dryness and irritation.

There are also creams or gels for vaginal use that you can only get on prescription. These contain small amounts of the female hormone oestrogen, which nourishes the lining of the vagina and makes it more moist. These include Vagifem, Ovestin, Premarin and Ortho-Gynest. There has been some concern that using a cream containing oestrogen might increase the risk of the cancer coming back in women who have had breast cancer. However, most experts believe that very little of the hormone is actually absorbed from the vagina and so there probably is no risk, but if you have had breast cancer it is best to check with your specialist before using one of these preparations.

Men may often find that getting an erection is more difficult while they are having chemotherapy and for some time afterward. This may have a variety of causes, which may be both emotional and physical. Anxiety and depression can both play a role here, and once again just talking about and understanding the problem may make a difference. Also, adjusting your love making to a pattern in which the man needs more time, encouragement and stimulation than before might make a difference. If depression is a problem then an antidepressant may help. If there is a more physical basis for the difficulty, as a result of either the treatment given or the effects of the cancer itself, then drugs like sildenafil (Viagra), vardenafil (Levitra) or tadalafil (Cialis) may help. These are only available on prescription, so you would need to discuss this with your doctor. Other solutions for physical problems include small injections of drugs such as papavarine or alprostadil (Caverject, Viridal), which you can be taught to give as injections directly into the penis or, in the case of alprostadil, as pellets inserted into the penis. Another approach is the use of vacuum pumps, which can be attached to the penis before intercourse to stimulate an erection. Sorting out the right approach to this problem can be difficult, and you probably need to talk to your doctor to get his or her advice on what can be done to help.

As mentioned above, depression can be a cause of loss of interest in sex at this time. Feeling low and depressed while you are having chemotherapy is very understandable. But for some people this tips over into clinical depression, which becomes a more constant problem in which your mood is low all the times, and nothing and nobody seems able to cheer you up – life just seems pointless and hopeless. A loss of sex drive is almost always part of the picture of clinical depression. If this describes the way you are feeling, then do discuss things with your family doctor or hospital specialist because there are very good drugs that can be given to treat clinical depression, and the benefits can often be rapid and dramatic. This is not a problem that you should suffer when such easy, safe and effective help is available.

Another physical factor that may influence your sex life is a change in your physical appearance or body image. This may be due to treatment you have had before chemotherapy, such as an operation like a mastectomy, where a breast has been removed, or a bowel surgery that has left you with a colostomy, or it may be the presence of a central line needed for your chemotherapy treatment.

Once again changes in body image affect everyone differently. Some people take them in their stride and feel that a change in their physical appearance has little or nothing to do with the real 'them'. At the other extreme some people feel completely devastated by the change. Similarly, the effect on partners can be very variable, with some feeling that a mere physical change has not altered the person they know and love, whereas others find the altered appearance more unsettling.

Talking is the key to adjusting to this situation. It is likely that even if you have concerns, your partner is going to be less affected than you are and will be able to offer you reassurance that 'you' are still the person they love and care for, and that any change in your appearance makes no difference to those feelings.

In terms of physical sexuality, you or your partner might at first find a physical change off-putting. It is likely that after talking about it, that feeling will lessen or disappear. But if it remains a tension, then it might be possible to get round it by adjusting the technique of your love making such that you hide the change, covering the area with a sheet, say, or keeping certain bits of clothing on during intercourse. Sometimes, these new ways of love making actually lead not only to a renewal of desire but an increase in enjoyment with the novelty of the new approaches to sex.

This section has tended to look at the problems with sexuality during and after chemotherapy. But although there will always be times when sex does not appeal, many people find that they can continue not only to have sex during their treatment but to carry on enjoying it. If you feel like it, then there is no reason at all why you should not go ahead and have some fun!

Friends and neighbours

Having cancer and chemotherapy can sometimes alter day-to-day relationships with friends and neighbours. Sometimes the changes can be for the better, sometimes for the worse. If there is a problem, then it usually comes down to communication, with either them not understanding your feelings or you not understanding theirs.

Everyone handles their cancer and its treatment differently. You may feel most comfortable by trying to keep things as much to yourself as possible, not troubling other people with your thoughts and feelings, and carrying on as near to normal as possible. If this is a positive way forward for you, it helps you to feel empowered and in control of your situation, and makes you feel stronger, then that is fine. But if you are simply trying to put a brave face on things because you don't want to burden other people, feeling that if you do so you will be letting yourself down or giving in, then think again. So often, sharing your worries and talking things through can be very helpful and supportive. Bringing anxieties and stresses into the open can make them seem far less troubling than bottling them up.

Similarly, friends and neighbours may feel uncertain about how to handle your situation. Should they rush in with offers of help? Should they ask you about how you are getting on, or should they avoid the subject and pretend that nothing is happening? They may worry that visiting you will make you tired or expose you to the risk of minor infections. They may even worry that they could 'catch' cancer from you (which, of course, can never happen).

At the end of the day it is down to you how you want to handle this situation. If you want to try and carry on as normally as possible, and feel that you cope best in that way, then let people know. Equally, if you are happy to talk about what is happening to you, if by sharing some or all of what you are going through makes life easier, then – again – let those around you know that you would welcome their questions and concerns. Alternatively, you may just want the practical support that they can give – help with the shopping, lifts to and from the hospital, and looking after the children once in a while – without the emotional involvement of talking about your thoughts and feelings. But however you want to deal with things, it will make life easier for them and, more importantly, for you if you let them know.

Letting them know might be something you find quite straightforward, or you might find it difficult and just another problem to deal with. If this is the case then getting your partner, or someone close to you in the family, to have a word with friends and neighbours for you could solve the problem.

9

Clinical trials

Enormous progress has been made in cancer chemotherapy over the past 50–60 years. Most of that progress has been due to developments in cytotoxic treatment, with the discovery of new drugs and a better understanding of the way to use them, but in breast cancer and prostate cancer improvements in hormonal treatments have also made an important contribution. As a result of these changes many more people are cured of their cancers than previously, and the cure rate continues to improve every year. Furthermore, countless numbers of people who have incurable cancer will now live much longer than could ever have been believed possible in the 1950s and 1960s as a result of the improvements in drug treatment for their illness.

New chemotherapy drugs are constantly appearing, and new combinations of existing drugs are being tested. These developments are exciting and promise much for the future. But a word of caution may not be out of place here. It seems that almost every week there is a newspaper report, a magazine article or a television story about some new major breakthrough in the drug treatment of cancer, with a novel compound producing wonderful results. But many of these offer the illusion of future hope rather than the reality of proven results. They often deal with the earliest stages of testing of a new drug, frequently when it has only been used in the laboratory and not on any patients at all, and then use these findings as the basis for all the excitement. Eager researchers, pharmaceutical companies with a vested interest, and even cancer charities anxious to attract publicity and donations will often encourage the media, who are always keen for stories, because cancer 'sells'. Before you know it, a first small step in the laboratory has become the new magic bullet for cancer.

All too often, anxious patients and concerned relatives and friends hear these reports and feel that if they cannot get the new drug then they must be missing out, that their chances of a cure or an increase in life expectancy are being jeopardized, when in reality there may be little or no evidence that the compound has any effect at all. At the same time, this pursuit of new, highly publicized treatments can often blind people to the fact that very active, good, tried and tested therapies already exist for their particular type of cancer, which can offer them an excellent chance of success.

So novelty is not everything. There is already a huge range of treatments that have proved their worth, and which are all freely available on the NHS for people with cancer.

Why do we need trials?

These days many people who are going to have chemotherapy will be offered the chance to take part in a clinical trial. Often the thought of being in a trial can be quite worrying, with feelings that you might be a guinea pig for the research of some mad scientist. But clinical trials are vital to the progress of cancer treatment, and nowadays there are so many safeguards for patients that you need not have any real anxieties.

Fifty years ago there were virtually no clinical trials. Doctors made their decisions about their patients' treatment based on their training and experience. Often those decisions were easy to make – if someone had appendicitis then you needed to operate to remove their appendix, if someone had pneumonia then you needed to give them antibiotics. But as more new treatments began to appear, it became more difficult to be sure which was the best to use in any particular situation. And so clinical trials were developed, so that treatments that seemed to be more or less equally effective for a particular condition could be compared to see whether one really was any better than the other.

In the 1960s the thalidomide disaster occurred, in which women were given that drug during early pregnancy to treat morning sickness. It was only later discovered that in many cases thalidomide caused damage to the growing embryo, leading to severe deformities of the limbs. This led to new rules about the testing of drugs before they could be used for routine treatment. Before thalidomide there had been very little done to make sure new drugs were safe when they were brought into use. Since thalidomide, all new drugs have had to go through careful trials or studies to make sure that their possible side effects are fully understood and that they can be used safely.

This means that there are broadly two types of clinical trial: those that are used in the early stages of a drug's development, to test its safety and effectiveness; and those that are used to compare new treatments – once they have proved to be safe and effective – with existing therapies to see whether they offer any advantage. The early trials are often called phase 1 and phase 2 trials, whereas the comparisons of treatments are called phase 3 trials.

Most people who have cancer and are offered trial entry will be asked whether they would like to take part in phase 3 studies. Usually, only people who have very advanced cancer, and who are no longer likely to be benefit from more established treatments, will be offered entry into the more experimental phase 1 and 2 studies, in which the value of the new treatment and its possible side effects are still uncertain.

Comparative (phase 3) clinical trials

Almost every week the newspapers report some new wonder drug for cancer treatment. These stories usually end with a sentence or two explaining that the results are at an early stage and that more testing will need to be done before the drug can be widely used. Unfortunately, the great majority of these 'wonder drugs' fail to pass the assessments of phase 1 and 2 trials, either proving ineffective or showing unacceptable toxicity. For the tiny handful of compounds that do successfully overcome these hurdles, the final test is the phase 3 comparison with the best of the currently available treatments.

There is a tendency to think that just because something is new, it will be better. But for many types of cancer there are well established and very effective therapies. So any novel drug must show that it has something to add to these, either by being better at treating the cancer, being just as good but having fewer side effects or offering some other benefit.

Phase 3 cancer clinical trials are carefully designed by teams of oncologists and statisticians. They produce a protocol – a document that sets out exactly what the trial is trying to discover and how it will be carried out. These protocols then have to be approved by panels of experts, who look at the scientific value of the work, and by an ethics committee, which includes lay members, to ensure that the study is safe and the well-being of people who take part in it is protected. So any phase 3 trial will have been very carefully checked before it is allowed to go ahead.

Usually, these trials will compare two or more different treatments for a particular type and stage of cancer. If doctors already have good evidence that one of these treatments is better than the others they would not need to do the study; these trials are done when the available results suggest that treatments are quite similar and more careful testing is needed to see whether one really is better than the others.

Sometimes a new treatment may become available for a condition in which there was no treatment on offer in the past. In this situation, if the merits of the new treatment are still uncertain, a trial may be done in which it is compared with an inactive compound, or placebo. In this way one group of people in the study will have a harmless but completely ineffective drug, which would be the same as the old situation of having no treatment, and be compared with the other people included in the trial who get the new active drug.

Most trials are designed in such a way that if once a particular treatment clearly shows a benefit over the other treatments being tested, then the study can be stopped, and everyone offered the most effective drug.

Nearly all of these comparative phase 3 trials will be randomized. This means that when someone goes into the study they will have the various treatment options explained to them but neither they nor their doctors will be able to choose which treatment they have. This choice will usually be made by a telephone call to the trial centre, where the treatment will be allocated according to a pattern predetermined by a computer. The reason for this is that if people were left to choose the treatment that they preferred or accept recommendations from their doctors, then this could influence the results of the study and lead to a bias in favour of a particular treatment, which would in turn lead to false results. So if you have already made up your mind what treatment you really want then taking part in a trial is probably not for you, because the final decision on what will be done is taken out of your hands.

If you are invited to take part in a clinical trial, then a number of things should happen.

- Your doctor should give you a full explanation of what is involved. This will often be backed up with a talk with a research doctor or nurse who is involved in running the study.
- You should receive written information in the form of a 'patient information sheet', giving you details of the study and what it will mean for you.
- You should be given time to think about whether you want to take part, and should never be asked to make an instant decision.
- You should be given the chance to ask any questions you have about the study.
- No one should ever put pressure on you to join a trial.

Often, taking part in a trial will mean that you have more hospital visits for check-ups and tests than normal. This is because of the various things that are being measured in the study and the need for very careful monitoring of how you are progressing. Some people like this and are glad of the extra care and attention involved, whereas others might find it inconvenient to have more appointments and investigations than are usually necessary. Once again, it pays to make sure you know what will be involved before you make a decision about whether to take part.

If you are offered the chance to take part in a trial and decide not to, this should not affect your future treatment or the care and attention you receive from your doctors and nurses in any way. They will respect your decision and will still continue to try to give you the best possible treatment and look after you just as well as if you were in the trial.

Overall, about one in ten people who have cancer will take part in a clinical trial at some time during their treatment, and these very often involve trials of different types of chemotherapy. For the past 40 years clinical trials have been the cornerstone for the improvement in the results of treatment with chemotherapy. There are many landmark studies that have resulted in better cure rates for numerous different types of cancer or years of extra life for people with advanced, incurable tumours, and many others that have brought improvements to people's quality of life by reducing the side effects of treatment.

10

Conclusion: what next?

You have reached the end of your treatment. It's over. The last blood test has been checked, the last drip has run through, you've swallowed your last anti-sickness tablet. You've made it – you heave a huge sigh of relief, and then ...? Perhaps surprisingly, for many people finishing chemotherapy can be a surprisingly difficult time. There are no more of the frequent trips to hospital, no more tests, no more drugs and no more side effects, but for the last few months all those sessions have provided a routine – a structure to life. And they have meant that you had got to know the nurses and doctors, and other members of the team who were looking after you. You had regular support, regular check-ups, and people to talk to about problems and concerns. But now you are on your own, and that can be hard. With so much progress in cancer treatment in recent years, more and more people are surviving cancer and finding that life after treatment can present problems, and cancer survivorship is now becoming a key issue (see *The Cancer Survivor's Handbook* by Dr Terry Priestman, Sheldon Press 2009).

You probably don't feel quite as well as you had expected. The sickness may have stopped, your hair may growing back and other things may be settling down, but you are still likely to feel pretty tired and are wondering how long that weariness will take to disappear.

You've got your next appointment with the specialist in a month or so, but that leaves a lot of time for you to wonder how things have gone, how successful your treatment has been and what the future holds. A whole range of thoughts, feelings and emotions that have been shelved or suppressed during the hurly burly of treatment can now surface, and often take you by surprise.

So be prepared for this to be a more difficult time than you had thought during all those weeks or months when you just couldn't wait for the day when it would all be over.

Half the battle in coping with this period is to realize that you might not find it as easy as you had expected. Be ready for the feelings of loss of contact with the hospital team and friends you had made during your time on treatment. Be ready for the fact that although the acutely upsetting side effects of treatment are over, there is still a background weariness that limits how much you can do. Be prepared for the questions and uncertainties about the future that will come crowding into your mind.

If you are lucky enough to have supportive, understanding family and friends, then this time will be easier. Chatting things through with people, who may do no more than just listen, can be very helpful. If you are on your own then it may be more difficult, but planning and enjoying a holiday, days out, or even just local visits and shopping trips can all provide a distraction and help fill the gap in life left by the end of your treatment.

For many people this becomes quite a spiritual period, not necessarily with a turn to conventional religion but still a time for personal reflection about life.

Being diagnosed with cancer, and going through a major treatment like chemotherapy because of that diagnosis, brings people face to face with questions of life and death. For many people it is a time to take stock of their life and its meaning. A time to look at where you want life to go in the future. A time to work out what is important to you.

You are likely to look back on your diagnosis and treatment – to wonder why it was you who got the cancer. You may feel, whatever your doctors and nurses have told you, that there were things in your life that contributed to you getting the illness, things that you want to change in the future. And your treatment, if it involved chemotherapy, will almost certainly have been a major event in your life. Some of that experience will have been positive, and some undoubtedly will have been negative, but at the end of the day you have come through it. You will in some ways be a different person, you will have faced up to and taken on challenges, handled situations you had never expected to encounter and – one way or another – worked your way through them. Making sense of it all will take time, but you will have learned a lot about yourself. Usually, the insights that come from this are positive, allowing you to realize that you can – that you did – deal with a situation that most people think of as a terrifying ordeal. You are likely to be emotionally stronger, with a justifiable pride in your achievement as a survivor of it all.

Your body may have been battered and drained by the therapies you have gone through, and your mind may still be reeling to cope with all the changes in your life and how to make sense of the future. You may feel that the whole experience has enriched your life, or you may feel confused, uncertain and even bitter that fate gave you the cancer in the first place. But the fact that you have worked your way through the trauma of being told you have cancer, and then journeyed through months of treatment, with all its demands and downsides, means that you have survived, you have coped. In fact, when all is said and done, you are really pretty amazing. You can look back at your progress with justifiable pride and take strength from your achievement to build for the future.

Useful addresses

Information about cancer, treatment for cancer and living with cancer

There are many organizations that offer help and advice to people with cancer, and a lot of these cover just one particular type of cancer. The short list that follows gives details of the main providers of general information, and they all give details of and have links to many other sources of help that you may find useful.

These organizations will also give you more ideas for further reading – many of them have regularly updated lists of books, booklets and other reading material.

Cancerbackup

For many years Cancerbackup has provided a comprehensive information service for patients. It offers a telephone helpline to specially trained cancer nurses, who can give advice on all aspects of cancer and its treatment. It also produces nearly 70 booklets and more than 200 fact sheets on all aspects of cancer. There are also more than 1,200 questions and answers about cancer on its website. (The website also has the texts of all the booklets and fact sheets, and links to many other useful organizations.) In 2008 Cancerbackup merged with Macmillan Cancer Support, and all of its information can now be accessed from the Macmillan website, or is available from Macmillan headquarters.

In addition to offering the Cancerbackup information service, Macmillan Cancer Support provides a number of publications on cancer, including a useful booklet on benefits and financial help for cancer patients (all listed on its website). The website also has useful information on various aspects of cancer, including a directory of local cancer support groups, and patients' stories about cancer.

Macmillan Cancer Support
89 Albert Embankment
London SE1 7UQ
Tel.: 020 7840 7840
Freephone Helpline: 0808 808 00 00
Website: www.macmillan.org.uk

Other organizations

Cancer Research UK
Angel Building
407 St John Street
London EC1V 4AD
Tel. (Supporter Services): 0300 123 1861
Tel. (Switchboard): 020 7242 0200
Website: www.cancerresearchuk.org

As well as funding research on cancer, this organization has a website (<www.cancerhelp.org.uk>) that gives information about different types of cancer and their treatment, as well as a comprehensive list of clinical trials currently in progress.

DIPEx
www.healthtalkonline.org

The initials stand for 'Database of individual patient experiences'. The website covers a number of different illnesses, but has an extensive section on cancer. This not only gives some background information on various types of cancer, but has lots of stories from people who have had cancer, and who have gone through chemotherapy.

Index